Praise for
Smart but Scattered Teens

"I was hooked from the first chapter! This book has opened my eyes to ways to foster my son's strengths, not just criticize his weaknesses. With all the issues we battle daily, it's easy to forget the power of the positive. I'm thrilled to have a specific plan of action for targeting the skills my son needs to do better in school and become more focused and responsible."
—*Kim L.*

"Executive skills are critical to success in life, but may be delayed in some teens and young adults—and parents are often at a loss for how to help. *Smart but Scattered Teens* is just what parents need. This is a highly useful guide for improving teens' executive skills and motivating them to use the skills they already have."
—*Patricia O. Quinn, MD, coauthor of* Ready for Take-Off:
Preparing Your Teen with ADHD or LD for College

"An absolute 'must read' for parents. Many detailed examples show you exactly how to teach your teenager the skills needed for success in school and beyond. The clever strategies for getting around teens' creative resistance to making changes are particularly helpful. I will recommend this gem of a book to all of the parents and adolescents I treat."
—*Arthur L. Robin, PhD, coauthor of* Your Defiant Teen

"Does your teen's behavior have you tearing out your hair in frustration? Quit nagging and use this wonderfully insightful and practical book to coach your 'smart but scattered' teen for personal, educational, and social success."
—*William Pfohl, PsyD, past president, International School
Psychology Association*

Smart but Scattered Teens

SMART but SCATTERED TEENS

The "Executive Skills" Program for Helping Teens Reach Their Potential

Richard Guare, PhD
Peg Dawson, EdD
Colin Guare

THE GUILFORD PRESS
New York   London

© 2013 The Guilford Press
A Division of Guilford Publications, Inc.
370 Seventh Avenue, Suite 1200, New York, NY 10001
www.guilford.com

The information in this volume is not intended as a substitute for consultation with healthcare professionals. Each individual's health concerns should be evaluated by a qualified professional.

Printed in the United States of America

This book is printed on acid-free paper.

Last digit is print number: 9 8 7 6 5

Library of Congress Cataloging-in-Publication Data

Guare, Richard.
    Smart but scattered teens : the "executive skills" program for helping teens reach their potential / Richard Guare, Peg Dawson, and Colin Guare.
        p.   cm.
    Includes bibliographical references and index.
    ISBN 978-1-60918-229-8 (pbk. : alk. paper) — ISBN 978-1-4625-0699-6 (hbk. : alk. paper)
    1. Parent and teenager.   2. Executive ability in adolescence.   3. Self-control
in adolescence.   4. Attention in adolescence.   5. Parenting.   I. Dawson, Peg.
II. Guare, Colin.   III. Title.
    HQ799.15.G83 2013
    306.874—dc23
                                                                    2012036449

Contents

PART III
Putting It All Together

Purchasers of this book may download copies of practical tools from *www.guilford.com/guare-forms.*

Authors' Note

In this book we have alternated between masculine and feminine pronouns to be inclusive; all information, anecdotes, and advice apply to both genders. The illustrations and stories in this book are all composites based on the problems and solutions we have seen over and over in our work and personal lives, and all names and personal details are fictitious. Several teenagers graciously shared their advice and other comments in Chapters 9–19. We have used the teenagers' own words, though their names have been changed to protect their privacy.

Introduction

Worrying about our teens comes with the job of parenting. We cross our fingers when they say good-bye on their way out the door on a Friday night, feel their frustration when they furrow their brows and agonize over schoolwork, wonder if they'll ever survive on their own when we spot a backpack sitting by the door, left behind and full of work that won't make it in on time without a parental delivery service. Parenting a teen through adolescence can be hard in the best of circumstances.

Yet for some parents the years from 14 to 19 are doubly difficult. If your teen can't seem to manage daily responsibilities or even minor problems, you undoubtedly find yourself worrying about these issues much more frequently than other parents. For you, the struggle to surmount your teen's ongoing problems, to strive to raise a self-sufficient, accountable adult, may feel like a never-ending battle.

You know your teen is smart enough, and sometimes you marvel at how really bright and creative your son or daughter can be. Just look at the things your teen can accomplish! So why is the morning routine still more chaotic than orderly? Why can't your teen seem to organize belongings and remember to take along whatever is needed for school, for a practice or a game, for a job or a college interview? Why are papers typically late, appointments missed (or never scheduled to begin with), the teen's room in disarray? Why do you have to hold your breath whenever your teen takes the car or has open-ended plans with friends?

Your teen is probably trying—and trying hard—to do everything his or her peers are expected to do as they mature and face increasing responsibilities. But it's a daily struggle when the teen has a deficiency in what are called *executive skills,* the functions of our brains and thought processes that help us regulate

1

our behavior, set goals and meet them, and balance demands and desires, wants, needs, and have-tos.

We've written this book to explain why your teen at one minute can seem so capable and at the next minute can't get out of his or her own way—to tell you that it's not a lack of smarts, or deliberate defiance, or just being a teenager. Even more important, we've written this book to give you strategies that can help—methods that have been shown to build the skills your teen lacks in full measure as well as tactics that will help your teen work around a weak skill and get the job done in a way that plays to the teen's strengths.

This may not be the first time you've had to deal with your teen's struggles. Perhaps even when your son or daughter was younger you had to be on top of the child all the time about one thing or another. If that's the case, you may already have benefited from the practical help in our first book, *Smart but Scattered*. Voluminous feedback has told us that these methods are as effective when used by parents as they've proven to be in our research and clinical work in schools and private practice. That was a major impetus for the writing of this book. Whether your child has been struggling for years or looked pretty capable in grade school, the child is a teen now, demanding independence and on the verge of adulthood. Your daughter is insistent about making her own decisions and has made it clear that she doesn't want you to meddle in her affairs. Your teenage son wants to run his own life. If your teenager can't do so, what's going to happen? Is your teen going to get hurt? Is your child going to fail? Are you going to have to help your son or daughter manage forever?

This book is dedicated to offering the same kinds of help and support we provided in our first book, but with a particular emphasis on the realities of adolescence. With ever-growing responsibilities, a relentless drive to become independent, and a lot more influence from the outside world, particularly peers, your teen can no longer rely so much on you for assistance. And you can no longer expect your teen to accept it as much, as often, or in as many domains of the teen's life as you may like.

Adolescence brings new challenges, as you know all too well. Neuroscientists tell us that even teens with good executive skills can struggle at times with the behaviors governed by executive skills. Their brains are going through a critical stage of development, and these executive skills are not yet securely anchored. That's what accounts for the Jekyll and Hyde behaviors of your teen. One minute your teen is cool, calm, and rational, and the next minute he's a screaming, irrational, emotional train wreck. If this is the typical teen, imagine the one with executive skills weaknesses—can't find anything ("Mom, where did *you* put my backpack?!"), doesn't watch the road, no sense that deadlines really do exist in the world, willing to try whatever his friends do. If you have a teen with executive skills weaknesses, it's like taking the typical teen and cranking up the volume—everything is louder, more intense, more *scattered*.

You may have helped your child in the past by using your own executive skills, your own fully developed frontal lobes, to help her learn and compensate. You helped her organize belongings and reminded her where to look when she couldn't find her jacket. You worked with her on her book report and reminded her (repeatedly!) to turn off the TV and attend to her homework. But now you need ways to help your teen without constant fights and that your teen can accept and still feel like she's in charge of her own life. Neuroscience research tells us that the adolescent brain is primed for the acquisition of new skills. Teens are driven to seek out new experiences, more intense social and emotional relationships, and, for better or worse, new risks. While it can be cause for worry, this new quest for independence presents teens with daily opportunities to use executive skills. And it presents you with the chance to help your teen improve these skills. But if your goal is to see your teen develop executive skills and become independent, your role as a parent must be quite different from what it has been until now. Your teen wants the chance to try out her ideas, make her own decisions. So part of your job will change from leading to following her lead. Now you'll work through negotiation and compromise and positive communication. You'll encourage her to set and follow her goals and offer help if she wants it, even if her goals don't always match yours.

Before you panic, let's be clear. You're not going to give up your role as parent. You will still have clear expectations for school and home, for standards of behavior and rules (about curfew, behavior with friends, drugs and alcohol, driving, etc.). And above all, your job, as it always has been, is to keep your teen in the game, protect him from catastrophic risks and failures. But this doesn't mean you protect the teen from all mistakes or failures. When these occur, you help the teen get up and dust himself off (if he won't accept your help) and encourage him to give it another try. Your role now is to be a facilitator, a catalyst, and not a tiger mom or dad.

At times you probably wish there were some magic bullet—a pill, a spell, a dietary supplement—that would infuse your teen with whatever executive skills he or she seems to lack. Wouldn't it be great if there were a fabulous new product that could meet your needs? "Exec-u-Spray!" screams the infomercial that runs through your mind. "Simply spray your teen every morning with this miracle remedy and watch your teen finish homework, remember to walk the dog, resolve conflicts with the grace of a diplomat, and maintain a spic-and-span bedroom and organized notebooks—and much, much more!" We'd all pay a lot for such a cure to ease our own worry and make life easier for the teens we care so much about. We know they can go far, and our fondest wish is to help them get there. That's what this book is all about. It will take effort and commitment, but we've given you lots of tips for boosting your success rate with our strategies by knowing your teen's strengths and weakness as well as your own, the way you two interact, and the personality traits you each bring to the task.

As you go through the ups and downs (and you will!), keep in mind that you want the same things—for your teen to become independent and manage successfully on her own. She won't get there if you hover, direct, make the decisions. You can provide support and maybe even suggestions if requested. Otherwise, unless she is going to hurt herself significantly in a physical or psychological way (a C on a test doesn't qualify), let her try. And if it doesn't come out as you expected or hoped, accept it and decide what you might do differently the next time. Try to avoid using the teen's mistakes as an opportunity to step in and take over or to make it an "I told you so" moment.

How to Use This Book

Part I answers questions about why teens can be smart and still so scattered. In Chapter 1 we define executive skills and explain and illustrate how they are used or not used by your teen. This is where you'll also find scientific information on how adolescent brain development helps to explain the mysteries of teenage behavior. Chapters 2 and 3 offer you an opportunity to take a closer look at your teen's executive skills profile and your own as well. Helping your teen build executive skills is a lot easier when you know what kind of fit you two have in executive skills. Do you both struggle with seeing a task through to the end? If so, you can use your empathy for your teen's problems to provide the most encouraging help and share the tactics that have helped you complete your own chores and projects. Or you can determine that you're not likely to be of much help here and seek assistance from someone who is strong in sustained attention—perhaps your teen's other parent or another trusted adult. Knowing where your respective strengths and weaknesses lie is an essential foundation for skill building, but because independence versus support can be tricky to negotiate, we also help you identify the behavioral style of your teen in Chapter 2 and your parenting style in Chapter 3. You'll gain a new understanding of how much help your teen tends to welcome and how you tend to interact with him so that you can see whether changes in your relationship could further your goal of promoting executive skill development.

Part II provides a foundation for enhancing and promoting the building and use of executive skills. Chapter 4 provides a set of principles to follow in deciding how to approach executive skills weaknesses in your teen. For example, is the skill something he can learn on his own, or does he need your help? If he does need your help, how do you balance the amount of support you provide and your desire to see him become independent? What factors determine whether your teen can accept suggestions and support from you? How much support does he need, how long does he need it, and how do you pull back without seeing him fail? The answers to these questions will allow you to gauge how to approach your teen.

In Chapters 5–7 we present a framework for the strategies that you'll use to address executive skills weaknesses with your teen. We've broken these down into three categories of intervention: (1) making adjustments in the environment to improve the fit between your teen and the situation or problem she faces; (2) working with your teen to support her in learning executive skills; (3) strategies to motivate your teen to use the executive skills that she has within her repertoire. If you have read *Smart but Scattered*, you'll be familiar with this framework. However, with teenagers, the specific types of strategies change significantly. For example, a key environmental modification is changing the way you approach and communicate with your child. In terms of teaching, your role shifts from giving instruction and providing close supervision to helping your teen learn by doing and relying more on the expertise of professionals to work with your teen. To motivate your teen, we've focused on how you can use the things she wants (license, phone, car, money, etc.) to help her engage her executive skills.

In Part III we offer strategies for targeting specific skills you've identified as weak in your teen. Prior to the chapters addressing each individual executive skill, Chapter 8 provides a set of guidelines for where and how to begin. This includes considerations such as beginning with one specific problem that, if resolved would have a positive effect on your teen's and perhaps the family's life. (A smoother morning routine would be an example.) This chapter will also help you decide on the type and proper level of support to offer your teen.

Chapters 9–19 then take you through each executive skill individually. We describe what the skill is, how it is manifested in teen behavior, and how you can assess your teen's strength or weakness in that skill in more detail than allowed by the Chapter 2 questionnaire. Typical situations that can arise with particular skills weaknesses are presented in the form of vignettes that capture the problem as well as the teen–parent interactions and reactions. This is followed by a brief question-and-answer section that expands upon the suggestions and solutions in the vignettes and also addresses other manifestations of a weakness in that executive skill. These chapters also benefit from candid quotes from teens who give their opinion on how to deal with various issues, tell us how they would react to the "interventions" described in the vignette, and remind us what it feels like to be a person between the ages of 14 and 19 who is struggling with the combined challenges of growing independence and lagging executive skills.

In Chapter 20 we discuss coaching, an intervention strategy that is well suited to the development of executive skills in teens who are open to participating in the process. The coach, typically a trusted adult or peer at school chosen by the teen, works with him on developing strategies to manage academic demands and behaviors that may be an impediment to the teen's goals. Coaching can diminish teen–parent conflict by eliminating the need for constant performance monitoring (and nagging) by the parent. This process also moves the teen toward increased independence and management of his school performance.

Chapter 21 addresses the next major transitions that your teen will embark on—high school to college and/or to a job and to more independent living, whether this means an apartment or a college dormitory. We've spelled out the potential pitfalls in these transitions and the strategies and questions you need to keep in mind in watching your teen take this major step toward independence.

We sincerely wish that we could offer you a no-hassle product like "Exec-u-spray." We hope we're giving you the next best thing. There is no easy way or shortcut to acquiring lagging or absent executive skills. Executive skills development requires considerable time and effort on the part of your teen and you. More than that, especially in adolescence, skill development requires you to understand teen behavior and know the strategies that will be most effective in helping your teen acquire these skills.

To be of the most help to your teen, you need to know how to motivate the teen to use these skills, how to create an environment that fosters skill development, and how to partner with your teen to help him or her learn these skills. Your goal—and ours—is nothing less than successful independent living as your teen moves into adulthood.

Part I

WHAT MAKES YOUR TEEN SMART BUT SCATTERED

1

....

Executive Skills and the Teen Brain

It is Tuesday morning at 6:30 A.M. in the Smith household. There is no indication to Mr. or Mrs. Smith that Jesse, their 15-year-old son, is stirring, although he was supposed to be up at 6:15, since his bus comes at 7:00. His mother knocks loudly on his door to remind him that he needs to get up immediately or he will be late. In a voice muffled by his pillow, Jesse mumbles, "Relax, Mom, I'll get there on time." Mrs. Smith sighs. If Jesse misses the bus, she will need to drive him and won't be able to get to work early as planned. Jesse emerges from his room at 6:40, grabs a bowl of cereal, and casually leafs through the sports pages. Every few minutes, his mother reminds him of the time, and he in turn reminds her that she needs to relax. Jesse does manage to get out the door and make the bus but calls 15 minutes later to tell his mother he forgot his lunch and his algebra book, which has his homework in it. He thinks it's on his desk. Could she drop it off on her way to work, before the end of his first period? His mother agrees because she knows Jesse already has missing assignments.

In the last 2 weeks, Jesse has missed his bus twice, forgotten his soccer equipment once, and been late with a major English paper. His teachers have said that Jesse needs to be more responsible for himself and more motivated and conscientious if he expects to go to college. They know he can do the work if he makes the effort, and they have recommended that his parents consider letting him suffer the consequences of low grades and detention to help motivate him. His parents aren't convinced. Over the past year and a half, since he entered high school, "natural consequences" have not had a significant impact on Jesse's time management, sense of time urgency, or organization.

9

Jesse did well in elementary school. He was a bit disorganized but typically got good grades, and his teachers noted how creative he was. In middle school, his parents had to provide increased support, but he still managed good marks, although his grades for study skills were weaker. Since starting high school, however, Jesse has struggled more. Whereas in middle school teachers used agenda books and checked them at regular intervals, in high school the student is expected to manage these tasks more independently, and Jesse seems increasingly overwhelmed.

Mr. and Mrs. Smith are realizing that while Jesse expresses a desire to be more independent (he said he set an alarm for this morning), they need to provide continuing and in some cases increased support. They don't mind doing that as long as there is some end in sight, but Jesse doesn't seem to be developing the skills he needs to manage the increasing demands of high school. Nor does he welcome their help as he used to. The more irritably he responds, the more conflict seems to characterize their relationship. Now his parents are losing sleep over what will happen when he turns 16 and can drive. And how about after that, when he's ready for college? He has the academic ability, but will he succeed without the parental and teacher support he's getting now? Like many parents, Mr. and Mrs. Smith have a sense that the clock is ticking. How can a young man who is bright and who expresses a desire and an intention to go to college be so scattered?

The problem for Jesse, as for many adolescents, is not one of intelligence. During elementary and even middle school, Jesse demonstrated the ability to do well in school. Around the house, his parents can see that he's bright and engaging, and they, like his teachers, have seen the spark of creativity. When it comes to smarts, adolescents like Jesse have plenty. What they lack, however, are some of the brain-based skills that we all need to plan and direct activities, to regulate behavior, and to make efficient and effective use of these smarts. The trouble does not show up in math or reading; rather, it shows up when they need to regulate their behavior to respond to the demands of a specific situation. Despite their good intentions, these adolescents can struggle with time management and organization. They can say things in conversation or take risks in situations where it seems like they should know better. They do not lack the intelligence to know better, but they may well lack the *executive skills* to help them use that intelligence to regulate their behavior.

What Are Executive Skills?

When people hear the term *executive skills,* they sometimes assume it refers to a set of skills required of good business executives—skills like strategic planning, decision making, and information management. There is some overlap—executive skills definitely include decision making, planning, and management of information, and, like the skills used by a business executive, executive skills help kids get done what needs to get done. But in fact, the term as we use it comes from the neurosciences literature and refers to brain-based skills required for humans to effectively execute, or perform, tasks and solve problems.

By the time your child has reached adolescence, she (like you) needs executive skills to manage the range of tasks and problems she will confront on a daily basis, as well as to regulate her behavior in the face of the temptations and distractions that will arise from the presence of peers. From activities as simple as getting up in the morning or remembering to take a homework assignment to school, to the complexity of managing school and extracurricular activities or driving in a car with a group of peers, executive skills are essential. For 15-year-old Jesse, managing his morning routine requires a number of executive skills. If the morning is to go smoothly and without the nagging of his parents, he needs to plan how much time he will need in the morning, remember to set his alarm clock, organize his homework and get it into his backpack, and get to sleep at a decent hour, inhibiting the urge to respond to the nearly continuous flow of text messages from his friends. If he does manage to remember to set his alarm, when it goes off in the morning he needs to initiate getting himself out of bed instead of opting for the immediate pleasure of additional sleep and then run through a mental checklist of what he needs to get together before he gets on the bus.

Let's be clear here. In general, many teens will have wake-up issues. These come with the territory of adolescence. From a biological perspective, the "wake–sleep clock" in adolescents' bodies changes so that they are naturally awake later but still need a good night's sleep. Unfortunately they live in a school world that does not accommodate these changes. School starts early, and even if nothing else were going on, waking up would be somewhat of a struggle. Add to that a day crammed with school, extracurricular activities, and socializing, and you get some idea of what keeps them up late at night. So even teens with good executive skills are going to struggle at times. Biology and busy lives conspire to ensure this.

Our point about Jesse is that when the system is taxed further by a weakness in executive skills, the struggle begins to take a significant toll on the teen's and parents' lives and threatens to impact school performance in a student who is more than academically capable.

For teenagers who struggle with these skills, more trouble lies ahead as the tasks in life become more complicated and more demanding of their ability to plan, sustain attention, organize information, and regulate feelings and how to act on them.

Executive skills are, in fact, what your teenager needs to make any of your hopes and dreams for her future—or her hopes and dreams—come true. By late adolescence, our children must meet one fundamental condition: they must function with a reasonable degree of independence. That does not mean that they do not ask for help and seek advice at times, but it does mean that they no longer rely on us to plan or organize their day for them, tell them when to start tasks, bring them items they've forgotten, or remind them to pay attention at school. When our children reach this point, for most of us our parenting role is coming to an end. We begin to speak of our children as being "on their own" and hopefully accept this at some level of comfort, as well as hoping for the best for them. Social institutions do the same, defining them as "adult" for most legal purposes.

To reach this stage of independence, a child must develop executive skills. You have probably seen an infant watch his mother leave the room, wait for a short time, and then begin to cry for his mother's return. Or maybe you have listened to your own 3-year-old telling herself (in a voice that sounds suspiciously like your own) not to do something. Or how about watching a 9-year-old who actually stops and looks before he races into the street after a ball? Or maybe you've watched your teenage son secure a job and take care of his work schedule without your assistance. In all of these cases, you are witnessing the development of executive skills.

Our Model

Our initial work in executive skills dates to the 1980s. While evaluating and treating children with traumatic brain injuries, we found deficits in executive skills to be the source of many cognitive, behavioral, and academic problems. In our clinic we also noted similar, although less severe, types of problems in children with attention disorders. From these origins, we began investigating the development of executive skills for a broad range of children and adults. While there are other systems for developing executive skills (the Resources section at the back of the book includes references for these systems), our model has been designed to achieve a specific goal: to help us come up with ways that parents and teachers can promote the development of executive skills in kids who have demonstrated weaknesses.

We based our model on two assumptions:

1. *Most individuals have an array of executive skills strengths as well as executive skills weaknesses.* In fact, we found that there seem to be common profiles of strengths and weaknesses. These patterns apply across the board to children and adults, for those who are developing typically as well as those who have been diagnosed with cognitive, behavioral, or academic difficulties. We wanted a model that would enable people to identify those patterns so that kids could be encouraged to draw on their strengths and work to overcome or bypass their weaknesses to improve overall functioning. We also found that it made sense to help parents identify their own strengths and weaknesses so they could be of the greatest help to their kids.

2. *The primary purpose of identifying areas of weakness is to be able to design and implement interventions to address those weaknesses.* We wanted to be able to help children build the skills they need or find ways to manipulate the environment to minimize or prevent the problems associated with the skill weaknesses. The more discrete the skills are, the easier it is to develop specific definitions of them. When the skills can be defined specifically, it is easier to create interventions to improve those skills. For example, let's take the term *scattered.* It is great for a book title because as parents we read the word and know immediately that it describes our child. But "scattered" could mean forgetful, disorganized, lacking persistence, or distracted. Each one of these problems would call for a different solution. So the more specific we can be in our problem definition, the more likely we are to come up with a strategy that actually solves the problem.

The scheme we arrived at consists of 11 skills:

- Response inhibition
- Working memory
- Emotional control
- Flexibility
- Sustained attention
- Task initiation
- Planning/prioritization
- Organization
- Time management
- Goal-directed persistence
- Metacognition

These skills can be organized in two different ways: developmentally (the order in which they develop in kids) and functionally (what they help the child do). Knowing the order in which these skills emerge during infancy, toddlerhood, and beyond, as mentioned earlier, can help you understand how your teenager arrived at the point where she is, as well as what you can expect from her as she moves through adolescence. While all executive skills are important, when it comes to teenagers, parents are likely to be particularly aware of the impact of specific skills. For example, in managing the demands of school, sports, work, and an active social life, the skills of planning/prioritization, organization, task initiation, and time management are particularly important. In terms of the types of activities that teenagers engage in that keep parents awake at night, they will want to know that their children have the capacity for response inhibition so that they do not routinely engage in impulsive and risky behaviors. And as driving comes into play, sustained attention becomes a critical skill. This is especially true since sustained attention can easily be affected negatively by one of the most important elements in a teenager's life, the presence of peers, as well as the constant availability of devices to maintain contact with those peers.

In the table on pages 15–17 are listed executive skills in the order of emergence, definitions of each skill, and examples of how they are manifested in teens.

When Do the Different Executive Skills Begin to Develop?

Infant research tells us that response inhibition, working memory, emotional control, and attention all develop early, in the first 6–12 months of life. We see the beginnings of planning a little later, when the child figures out a way to get a desired object. Flexibility shows in the child's reaction to change and can be seen between 12 and 24 months. The other skills, such as task initiation, organization, time management, and goal-directed persistence, come later, ranging from preschool to elementary school, with metacognition coming latest, at 10 or 11 years of age.

In some cases, parents know well before adolescence that their children have weaknesses in executive skills. A problem with flexibility might show up in preschool as regular tantrums in response to unexpected change. You might have learned early on that it was important to maintain predictable routines for your child. As time went on, the foot-stomping tantrums may have subsided, but you still recognize the burst of anger in your teen when you present an agenda

Definition and Examples of Executive Skills

Executive skill	Definition	Examples
Response inhibition	The capacity to think before you act—this ability to resist the urge to say or do something allows your child the time to evaluate the situation and how his behavior might impact it.	Some teenagers think about the consequences before they do something. Other kids just act—they don't waste time thinking about the consequences.
Working memory	The ability to hold information in memory while performing complex tasks. It incorporates the ability to draw on past learning or experience to apply to the situation at hand or to project into the future.	Some kids keep track of their belongings, like coats, keys, or sports equipment, or are really good at remembering what they have to do. Other kids forget where they have left stuff and misplace things a lot or say, "I'll do it later," but then forget about it. Some kids seem to learn from experience; others don't.
Emotional control	The ability to manage emotions to achieve goals, complete tasks, or control and direct behavior.	Some teenagers have a short fuse and get easily frustrated by little things or get stressed out if something doesn't go right. Other teenagers can stay cool despite irritation and take unexpected events in stride.
Flexibility	The ability to revise plans in the face of obstacles, setbacks, new information, or mistakes. It relates to an adaptability to changing conditions.	Some teenagers can "go with the flow" and adjust fairly easily to a change in plans. Others plan out in their head in advance how something will go and get upset if it doesn't happen as planned.
Sustained attention	The capacity to keep paying attention to a situation or task in spite of distractibility, fatigue, or boredom.	Some kids complete homework or chores without having to be hassled by their parents, while other kids start but don't finish unless someone is on their case.

Executive skill	Definition	Examples
Task initiation	The ability to begin projects without undue procrastination, in an efficient or timely fashion.	Some kids are good at making themselves set aside fun stuff to do their homework or to start on their homework right away. Other kids have a hard time pulling themselves away from fun things (texting, Facebook) to do work and put off homework as long as possible.
Planning/ prioritization	The ability to create a road map to reach a goal or to complete a task. It also involves being able to make decisions about what is important to focus on and what is not important.	Some kids are good at figuring out the steps needed to do a project or figuring ways to save money for something they want. Others don't know where to start or how to make a plan, or want expensive things but don't know how to go about saving money for them.
Organization	The ability to create and maintain systems to keep track of information or materials.	Some kids keep notebooks and backpacks organized to find things easily or put things back in a specific place as soon as they have finished using them. Other kids can't find things in their notebooks or backpacks because they are a mess, or they leave their belongings around the house (or even at other people's houses!).
Time management	The capacity to estimate how much time one has, how to allocate it, and how to stay within time limits and deadlines. It also involves a sense that time is important.	Some kids are reliably on time for school or can finish their homework in the time that they have available. Other kids are chronically late or routinely scrambling to make a deadline, or always seem to run out of time for the homework they have to do.

Executive skill	Definition	Examples
Goal-directed persistence	The capacity to have a goal, follow through to the completion of that goal, and not be put off or distracted by competing interests.	Some kids are willing to set aside fun stuff to achieve a long-term goal or find ways around the obstacles that might stand in the way of getting what they want. Other kids live by the precept "You're only young once" or give up working toward a goal if something blocks them.
Metacognition	The ability to stand back and take a bird's-eye view of yourself in a situation, to observe how you problem-solve. It also includes self-monitoring and self-evaluative skills (for example, asking yourself, "How am I doing?" or "How did I do?").	Some kids are good at sensing how others are reacting to their behavior or ideas. Other kids focus more on getting their point across and may not pick up on feedback from others.

different from the one he was planning. If your child's kindergarten teacher reported that your child couldn't wait his turn, was constantly out of his seat, and spoke without raising his hand, you might have been observing weak response inhibition. In adolescence, this weakness might evolve into fooling around and talking out in class and, on the home front, risk taking, particularly behind the wheel. (This is Dick talking:) When I volunteered in my son's first-grade class, I saw him regularly daydream through teacher directions, and throughout elementary school I was a regular visitor to lost and found. Interestingly, I often saw the other parents whose kids struggled with these skills there, and we came to recognize the belongings of one another's children, at times dropping them off for each other. Car keys, books, cell phones, and articles of clothing all fell victim to his weaknesses with attention and organization when he was a teenager.

If you've been seeing problems like these since your teen was younger, chances are you've developed some strategies and probably teaching techniques so you and your child could cope better with these situations. Interventions like maintaining predictable routines, designating when he could have his turn, and establishing a place for belongings and cues to put them there are all strategies that parents can use effectively. During adolescence, the principles that guide the earlier interventions (change the environment, teach the skill, motivate the teen to use the skill) don't change. What does change is the approach (moving from giving a direction to conducting a negotiation) and the situations around which the negotiations occur. Much of the remainder of this book is devoted to spelling out the details of these interventions for you.

On the other hand, your experience could have been with a teen more like Jesse. That is, perhaps you haven't seen significant problems before now. This is likely because the supports provided by you and by the school were sufficient to prop up your teen's weak skills. With time, as a child ages and moves into middle and then high school, expectations change ("They need to be more responsible for themselves"), and family and institutional supports gradually fall away. For these children, increasing demands on executive skills coupled with a decrease in naturally occurring supports expose a problem that may not have required significant intervention in the past.

Thinking Skills versus Doing Skills

Knowing how each skill functions—whether it contributes to teenagers' thinking or doing—tells you whether the goal of your intervention is to help your child think differently or to help your child behave differently. If your adolescent has weak working memory, for instance, you will be working with her on strategies to help her retrieve critical information (such as what she has for specific homework assignments). If your teenager has weak emotional control, you will be working with him on strategies to control his temper when he finds out that his little brother has removed something from his room. In fact, though, thinking and doing go hand in hand. Very often, we are teaching kids how to use their thoughts to control their behaviors.

Thinking skills are designed to select and achieve goals or to develop solutions to problems. They are especially important skills for teenagers because they help them create a picture of a goal and a path to that goal, and they give them the resources they will need to access along the way to achieve that goal. They also help the teenager remember the picture, even though the goal may be far away, when other events come along to occupy his attention and take up space in his memory. But to reach the goal, your teenager needs to use the second set of skills, ones that enable him to do what he needs to do to accomplish the tasks he sets for himself. This second set of skills incorporates behaviors that guide the teenager's actions as he moves along the path. The organizing scheme is depicted in the table below.

When all goes as planned, beginning in early childhood, we come up with ideas for things we want or need to do, plan or organize the task, squelch the thoughts or feelings that interfere with our plans, cheer ourselves on, keep the goal in mind even when obstacles, distractions, or temptations arise, change course as the situation requires, and persist with our efforts until the goal is achieved. This may be as time-limited as completing a 10-piece puzzle or as extensive as remodeling our house. Whether we are 3 years old or 30, we rely on the same set of brain-based skills to help us reach our goal.

Developmental Trends

As you've watched your child grow and develop, you've seen changes and improvements in your child's ability to regulate her behavior, in other words, in her executive skills. While at 2 years old you wouldn't have thought of letting go of your child's hand in a busy parking lot, by age 7 you may well have been comfortable with her walking independently, relying only occasionally on verbal reminders. From the time of our children's first independent movements, in the first year of life, we are increasingly aware of their ability and desire for

Two Dimensions of Executive Skills: Thinking and Doing

Executive skills involving *thinking* (cognition)	Executive skills involving *doing* (behavior)
Working memory	Response inhibition
Planning/prioritization	Emotional control
Organization	Sustained attention
Time management	Task initiation
Metacognition	Goal-directed persistence
	Flexibility

independence. At the same time, we are aware that their executive skills are not well enough developed for the children to manage their behaviors or solve problems without direction or guidance from us. Everything we teach our children reflects our understanding of how we are using our executive skills to help them develop and refine their executive skills.

Now, as our children enter adolescence, we become acutely aware of how important this skill development has been and will continue to be if our children are to safely negotiate the challenges of adolescence and emerge in 4 to 6 years with sufficient ability to manage on their own. Understanding their skills and the support that we need to provide during this period is especially critical for a number of reasons. As a natural part of development, teenagers want to establish their own identity. From the teen's perspective, a key feature of establishing one's identity is the ability to make decisions independently. A second significant feature of adolescence is the increased influence of peers on the teenager's decision making and the corresponding decrease in parents' influence. The third critical element in this period is the fact that there are real challenges and potential risks associated with these decisions in the teenager's world. These challenges include managing school demands, establishing positive social interactions with peers, and maintaining safety in the context of driving, availability of alcohol and drugs, and the beginning of sexual relationships.

Parents of teenagers, particularly of those children with weak executive skills, face their own set of challenges during this period. On the one hand, most parents recognize that they must continue to provide guidance for their children to avoid serious, if not catastrophic, mistakes. On the other hand, they recognize that their children will show various degrees of resistance to this guidance. For those parents who attempt to control their child's decision making, there is likely to be frequent conflict. When parents avoid providing this guidance, the likelihood of poor decision making on the part of the teen is increased significantly. Before we get into how parents and teens can negotiate these challenges, it will be helpful for you to understand how children come by executive skills.

How Executive Skills Develop in the Brain: Biology and Experience

As is the case with many of our abilities, there are two main contributors to the development of executive skills—biology and experience. In terms of the

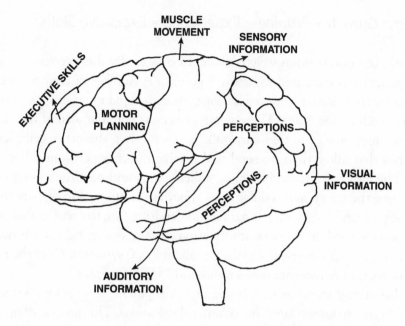

MUSCLE
MOVEMENT
SENSORY
INFORMATION
EXECUTIVE SKILLS
MOTOR
PLANNING
PERCEPTIONS
VISUAL
INFORMATION
PERCEPTIONS
AUDITORY
INFORMATION

The human brain, with the approximate location of major functions.

biological or neurological contribution, the potential for executive skills is essentially innate, already a part of the brain's wiring at birth. This is similar to the manner in which language develops. Naturally at birth, executive skills, like language, exist only as potential. That means that the brain has within it the basic biological equipment for these skills to develop, but a number of factors can influence how these skills develop. Any type of major trauma or physical insult to the child's brain, particularly if this involves the frontal lobes, will adversely affect executive skill development. Genes also can play a major role, and therefore the genes that the child inherits from you can also impact these skills. If you don't have good organizational skills or attention, there is a better chance that your child will have problems in these areas as well. As far as the environment is concerned, if it is biologically or physically toxic, there is an increased likelihood that the child's executive skills will suffer as a result. Environmental toxins can include anything from lead exposure to child abuse. And there is growing evidence that severe psychosocial stress can adversely impact executive skills development. However, if we assume reasonably normal biological equipment and the absence of genetic or environmental traumas, brain development will proceed as it is supposed to.

Biology: Growth + Pruning + Experience = Executive Skills

At birth, the child's brain weighs about 13 ounces. By the late teenage years, brain weight has increased to nearly 3 pounds. A number of changes account for this increase in size and weight. First, there is rapid growth in the number of nerve cells in the brain. These nerve cells must communicate if the child is to think, feel, or act. So they can "talk" to each other, the nerve cells develop branches that allow them to send and receive information from other nerve cells. The growth of these branches, called axons and dendrites, is especially fast during the infant and toddler years. They are connected to one another by synapses, which along with the axons and dendrites, are the wiring that allows our brains to send and receive information. In a newborn baby, each neuron, the cell that sends electrical signals, has about 2,500 synapses. Over the next 3 years or so, that number increases to around 15,000 synapses.

Also during these earliest stages of development, a substance known as myelin begins to form a fatty sheath around the axons. This process of myelination insulates the branches that carry the nerve impulses, making the "conversations" between nerve cells faster and more efficient. Myelination continues well into the late stages of adolescence and early adulthood and is responsible for the development of what is often called the white matter of the brain. The white matter consists of bundles of axons that connect different brain regions and allow them to communicate. Then there is gray matter. This is a term often used as a metaphor for the learning, thinking part of the brain itself. The reason for this is that gray matter is made up of nerve cells, or neurons, as well as synapses, the connections between them discussed above. The development of this type of brain matter is a bit more complex. At the fifth month of pregnancy, the brain of the unborn child is estimated to have about one hundred billion neurons. This is actually comparable to what the average adult brain has. Early in childhood, the total number of synapses in the brain (about a quadrillion) greatly exceeds the number there will be in the adult brain. If the development of neurons and gray matter continued at this pace, the adult brain would be enormous. Instead, a different phenomenon occurs. The increase in gray matter—neurons and particularly synapses—peaks before the age of 5 and is followed by a gradual reduction or "pruning" of the neuron connections. The initial increase happens during a period of rapid learning and experience in early childhood. Recent brain research suggests that as this learning and skill developmental become more efficient, additional increases in gray matter could actually undermine the learning.

Through pruning, the child consolidates mental skills, and the gray matter connections that are not needed or used drop away. Until recently, scientists thought this surge in neuron and synapse growth, followed by pruning, happened only once during child development, when children were young. However, recent research has demonstrated that there is another major surge in growth of neurons and synapses just before adolescence, followed by a process of pruning that extends throughout adolescence.

In terms of what we know about the development of executive skills, research shows that this growth spurt in the brain prior to adolescence occurs primarily in the frontal lobes. Scientists now generally agree that the frontal brain systems play a key, though not exclusive, role in the development of executive skills. Therefore, we can safely say that these areas, which include the frontal and prefrontal cortex, along with connections to adjacent areas, in large part make up the brain base for executive skills. As far as the growth spurt is concerned, it is as if during the preteen years the brain is preparing itself for the development of executive skills and the significant demands that will be made on those executive skills during adolescence. The diagram on page 21 shows the human brain with the approximate location of major functions, including executive skills, in the prefrontal cortex.

As part of this research looking at brain development during adolescence, scientists at the National Institute of Mental Health have also suggested that a "use it or lose it" process may be occurring in the frontal lobes during this time. Neural connections, including synapses, that are used are retained, while those that are not exercised are lost. If this is in fact the case, it means that the practice of executive skills is critical. Teenagers who practice executive skills are not only learning self-management and independence, but in the process are also developing brain structures that will support their executive skills into later adolescence and adulthood.

As noted earlier, you may have noticed executive skills weaknesses in your child early on and have been practicing these skills with her for some years. Does that put you ahead of the game? In the sense that you understand how the weaknesses manifest themselves and what strategies might work to help your teen be more successful, the answer is yes. Is your child in better shape to enter adolescence than the one whose parents are just now recognizing a weakness? Maybe. While earlier practice may have helped, you might have become aware of the problem earlier because the skill deficit was more significant. In that case challenges will still be significant in adolescence. Earlier practice has probably promoted the development of neural pathways underlying these skills, but continued practice will be essential if your teen is to manage the new executive skills demands that inevitably come with adolescence.

What about the teen who is showing problems for the first time? Is it too late to intervene? The answer is an emphatic no! In fact, the developing teen brain presents an excellent opportunity for you to influence executive skills in your teen. But to take full advantage of that opportunity you should be aware of certain reactions you and your teen may have that could throw up a roadblock. The realization that your teen is struggling and may need increased support can feel discouraging. For your teen, this struggle may feel humiliating—or at least acknowledging it probably feels like an impediment to the teen's desire for autonomy.

The key is understanding these factors, understanding the issue of weak or lagging executive skills, and knowing how to intervene using the resources we've provided here. This time period represents a critical window of opportunity for the practice and development of executive skills, so it's worth trying to overcome obstacles. To help you in this process, we have provided detailed guidelines for gauging how your teen responds to the problem and what approach will be most effective.

Practice is important to the acquisition of executive skills for another reason. Researchers who studied the brain using fMRI (functional magnetic resonance imaging) have found that when children and teenagers perform tasks that require executive skills, they rely on the prefrontal cortex to do nearly all of the work rather than distributing that workload to other specialized regions of the brain. Two of these other regions, the amygdala and the insula, are parts of the brain that are activated when making quick decisions that affect safety and survival (the fight-or-flight response). In contrast to children and teenagers, adults can spread out the workload in part because they have had years of practice to develop the neural pathways to make this possible. Activating executive skills takes more conscious effort with children and teenagers than it does with adults, which may help explain why they are less inclined to engage their executive skills to perform tasks of daily living. Related to this, recent research has demonstrated that when risky situations are described to adults, the risk is so obvious to them and they are so practiced at understanding the risks that they don't have to engage large areas of their frontal lobes. In contrast, the riskiness of a situation is significantly less obvious to adolescents, and they have to make an effort to engage the frontal lobes to determine if in fact the situation does represent a significant risk. Considering this, it is not hard to imagine that a group of teenagers challenging or encouraging one another to engage in a risky behavior can readily lead to bypassing this effortful thinking and impulsively engaging in the behavior. To highlight these issues of development in the adolescent brain, a recent article in *Parade* magazine compared the teenage brain to a Ferrari. It is fast, shiny, sleek, and it handles well. The problem is it has lousy brakes.

This is where you and your teenager's teachers, coaches, and employers come in. Adolescence offers parents and other adults in their lives a critical opportunity to enhance the development of executive skills in the teen. In the adolescent brain, the huge surge in brain wiring and the process of pruning these connections will extend into young adulthood. The biological changes occurring during this period represent the last significant alterations in the brain before it achieves mature adult status in the mid- to late 20s.

The Mystery of the Adolescent Brain—and Teenage Behavior

In one sense, the adolescent brain is well suited for the task at hand—learning the skills that will be required for adult living. Through practice and experience, the pruning process will continue and the brain will gradually shed unused synapses and dendritic branches, strengthen other synapses, and increase the efficiency of nerve transmission through myelination of axons. Over a period of 10 to 12 years, beginning around puberty, the plasticity of the adolescent brain allows for rewiring. What the final wiring diagram looks like depends on two factors: what teens bring with them up to puberty and what experiences they have over the next 10 years or so. While on the one hand adolescents have a brain that is primed for learning through experience, they also have a brain that is ill suited for fully independent decision making about what those experiences should be. Why? Let's consider some other characteristics of the adolescent brain. Above, we mentioned risk taking and noted that teens take more effort to engage their frontal lobes when considering risk. Nonetheless, when they do, their assessment of the degree of risk in a hypothetical situation is comparable to that of adults. Why is it, then, that they still engage in risky behavior more often than adults? It's because of what neuroscientists refer to as "hot" versus "cool" cognition. "Hot" cognition means that teens are thinking under conditions of intense emotion and high arousal (like when you and your teen disagree about an overnight beach party). You see the risk, but your teen sees the reward. For teens, anything that arouses emotion—fear of social rejection, the need to look cool, disappointing someone, disagreements with parents—can lead to "hot" (and less rational) thinking. This helps us understand why at times our children seem like mature, reasonable teens and at other times like moody, demanding 5-year-olds. It also explains why it is important for parents to maintain their "cool" in discussions and disagreements with teens. Strong emotional reactions from parents fuel the emotional reactions of teens.

A second characteristic of adolescent brains that can help us understand their behavior has to do with neurotransmitters. Neurotransmitters are chemical-like substances that travel between nerve cells across a synapse and determine whether a nerve signal keeps going or halts. Levels of two of these neurotransmitters, dopamine and serotonin, decrease during adolescence. The decrease in dopamine results in mood changes and problems with emotional control. The decrease in serotonin results in decreased impulse control. A third neurotransmitter, melatonin, increases in adolescence. Melatonin is responsible for circadian rhythms and the sleep–wake cycle. Its increase results in a need for greater sleep. This helps to explain how teens can sleep for extended periods on weekends. The increase also means that teens will be sleep deprived through the combination of staying up later, leading busy lives, and attending the early classes that we noted above. So we have "hot" thinking, increased moodiness, decreased emotional and impulse control, and fatigue, all of which come with the territory of adolescence.

A third facet of the adolescent brain involves a part of the brain called the limbic system, which is referred to as the more primitive or emotional part of the brain. As adults, we still experience the emotions and drives that originate from the limbic system, but the prefrontal cortex helps to regulate and "damp down" these emotions and drives. For teens, the incomplete development of the frontal lobes and prefrontal cortex, along with the changes noted above, means that they will rely more on the emotional parts of their brain in decision making. The result? They will be quicker to anger, show more intense mood swings, and make choices based on gut feelings rather than logic.

The final factor involves sensation seeking. The nucleus accumbens has been identified as one of the "reward centers" in the brain. This area of the brain is highly sensitive in teens, and it sends them powerful signals to pursue a desirable activity or situation. The neurotransmitter dopamine produces pleasurable feelings, but because teens have less dopamine available they will need more intense levels of stimulation to produce the same feelings of pleasure and reward. The result is that they will seek the excitement associated with new, more intense experiences and the thrill associated with risks.

How these four factors play out with any particular teen depends on his or her emotional makeup and vulnerabilities, state of frontal lobe development (in behavioral terms, how mature the teen is), and experience (does the teen feel competent in some area—social, academics, work, sports, arts?). Think of changes in the adolescent brain as "turning up the volume," particularly on whatever executive skills weaknesses and emotional vulnerabilities the teen brings into adolescence.

The All-Important Prefrontal Brain System

As we have noted above, the prefrontal brain systems play a key role in the development and application of executive skills. The prefrontal systems are among the last areas of the brain to develop fully, in young adulthood, and are the final, common pathway for how we manage information and how we regulate our behavior. As the frontal lobes develop, if they are working well, they help us manage our behavior and use our executive skills in the following ways:

1. The frontal lobes direct our behavior, helping us decide what we should pay attention to and what actions we should take. *Example:* A 17-year-old gets a text message from his friend inviting him to play an online video game that is starting in a few minutes. He wants to play but decides to finish his math homework, which he knows his mom will ask him about when she gets home.

2. The frontal lobes link our behaviors together so that we can use past experience to guide our behavior and help us make future decisions. *Example:* A 16-year-old remembers that when she has a plan to stay over with friends, her parents want details about the plan, including who will be there, what parent will be there, and contact information and a time when they can speak to that parent. Prior to asking her parents' permission, she prepares all of this information, including when and at what number they can contact her friend's parent.

3. The frontal lobes help us control our emotions and our behavior, taking into account external and internal constraints as we work to satisfy our needs and desires. By regulating our emotions and social interactions, the frontal lobes help us meet our needs without causing problems for ourselves or others. *Example:* A 15-year-old wants to attend a beach party with some new kids he has met at school. His 17-year-old brother informs his parents that there will likely be alcohol and drugs at the party. Although upset, the 15-year-old does not get into a fight with his parents or brother about the decision that he cannot go.

4. The frontal lobes help us observe, assess, and fine-tune, allowing us to correct our behavior or to choose a new strategy based on feedback. *Example:* A 16-year-old forgets her basketball jersey for a game and, as a result, is not allowed to play. She remembers to organize all of her equipment and check it before she leaves for school in the morning so that this will not happen again.

So in terms of biology and brain development, what does this mean for your teenager? First, we know that executive skills are critical to successfully negotiating the challenges of adolescence, including risk assessment and independent living. As parents, these are basic goals that we have for our children. Second, we know that at birth, executive skills exist only as potential; a newborn has no actual executive skills. Third, frontal brain systems, and therefore executive skills, will require approximately 25 years to develop fully. Given these factors, children and adolescents cannot rely solely on their own frontal lobes and executive skills to regulate behavior. What's the solution? We lend them our frontal lobes, acting as surrogate frontal lobes for our children. Although we might not think of it in these terms, parenting is, among other things, a process of providing executive skills support and coaching for our children. As we will see, for parents and their teenagers this is both critical and challenging.

Experience: Lending Your Child Your Frontal Lobes

In the earliest stages of your child's life, you simply were the frontal lobes for your child, and your child had little to contribute. Your own executive skills planned and organized your child's environment to ensure safety and comfort, monitoring of basic behaviors such as sleeping and eating, social interactions, and problem solving when your child was upset or distressed. Your child, as a newborn, had very few behaviors—sleeping, eating, crying—with which to manage her world and was totally dependent on your responses to her needs. But at about 5 or 6 months of age, your infant began to develop some of the skills that would eventually lead to self-management and independence. The first of these skills to develop, at about 5 or 6 months, was response inhibition. This ability to respond or not respond to a person or to a situation is at the heart of behavioral self-regulation. We are well aware of the trouble that our children can get into if they act before thinking. You may have been impressed in the past by the self-control of a child who could see a tempting object and not immediately touch or take it, and you'd be impressed now if you saw your teenager forgo meeting with friends to work on a school project. When your child began to develop this skill at about 6 months, you wouldn't have initially seen any striking changes. What you probably did note was that the infant was somewhat more active and interactive. Between 6 and 12 months, the baby's ability to inhibit or initiate responses grew significantly. For example, you might have seen your 9-month-old crawling toward her mom in the next room. Whereas a month or two earlier she might have been distracted by finding a favorite toy along the way, by 9 months she was crawling right past the toy on her way to her mother. You may also have noticed that your baby could now withhold some kinds of expression and show others depending on the situation. We have probably all had the experience of trying to engage a baby at this age who then doesn't respond at all or even turns away. It feels like rejection, doesn't it? Even at this young age, a baby is beginning to learn the powerful effect of responding or not responding to a particular person or situation. The 3- or 4-year-old shows this skill by "using his words" instead of hitting a playmate who tries to grab his toy. The 9-year-old is using the same response inhibition skill when he looks before running into the street to get a ball, and the 17-year-old shows response inhibition by staying near the speed limit instead of responding to his friend's suggestion "Let's see what this thing can do."

A second key skill developing in the same time frame is working memory. During the first 5 or 6 months of life, your infant lived perpetually in the present. If she couldn't immediately taste it, touch it, smell it, hear it, or see it, it did not exist. For the young infant, out of sight is out of mind. At about 6 months of age, your baby developed a very basic capacity to hold visual information (objects, places, people) in mind when not in its presence. This was the beginning of the child's being able to carry part of her world and her experience with her. This allowed for the chance to make choices and "decisions." For example, if Mom left and did not come back immediately, the baby could look to the last place where she saw her and cry. Mom might have returned. If this happened, the baby "understood" at some level that "If Mom leaves and I want her back, she will come if I cry."

As information and experience grew, working memory allowed your child to recall a past event, apply it to a present situation, and predict what might happen in the future. For example, suppose your child is now 15 years old. She might say to herself, "Last Saturday, after I helped with cleaning the house, Mom and I went shopping. I'll ask her if we can do something like that again after I help her with chores today." Or the 17-year-old could say, "My boss asked me to work tomorrow night. I need to tell her that I can't. The last time I

worked before a test, I didn't leave enough time to study and got a bad grade."
It is obvious that the baby's recall of Mom leaving the room was a far cry from
her skills at age 15 or 17, but with her ability to hold a picture of Mom in mind,
we can see the beginning of this control. To help our children develop a skill
like working memory, we provide them with certain types of experience. For
example, we provide manipulative "cause–effect" toys such that when the baby
performs an action, like banging it, the toy does something, like move or make
a noise, or we make toys "disappear" and have our children look for them. Once
the child can move, we might have him retrieve or search for objects. As he
gains language, the child begins to manage his behavior by remembering directions and rules repeated and displayed by you, and then later again, you can ask
questions like "What do you need for this activity?" or "What did you do the
last time this happened?"

In combination with response inhibition, we can begin to see how experience stored in working memory can influence the child's decision to respond or
not respond to a situation.

Throughout childhood, we see first these and then the other executive
skills beginning to emerge and develop so that by the time our children reach
adolescence, they are using all of these skills. At the same time, we are acutely
aware that these skills are not fully developed and that our children need the
continuing support of our frontal lobes to negotiate turbulence and manage
risks. Maybe you have a daughter who habitually leaves lit candles in her room
when she goes out for the night. Or your son has a penchant for lighting small
fires without a permit or a whole lot of common sense. Perhaps you know a teen
who never puts money in the meter and shoves parking tickets under the front
passenger seat. We know one teen who, on three separate occasions, has gotten
out of his car only to have it roll away, later blaming the fact that he left it in
gear while on an important phone call. We also know a high school sophomore
who tried to arrange a nighttime beach party with no chaperones.

As we have noted, these risks loom large for parents: driving, availability
of alcohol and drugs, and sexual relationships. In addition, we understand the
implications of poor school performance and the limits this can place on the
adolescent's options and choices at the end of high school. We can see the challenges, and we understand that our children do not always appreciate the longer-term consequences of their actions. In their day-to-day activities, they are
often what Russell Barkley describes as "context-dependent." By this he means
that their behavior is influenced largely by what they experience right here,
right now. Therefore, they are attracted to situations and activities that are fun,
interesting to them, and immediately rewarding (TV, video games, computer,

etc.). This characteristic of context-dependent behavior, along with the importance and influence of peers, keeps their focus in the present and makes it much more difficult for them to see what their behavior might mean for their future.

It is a Sunday morning in November. After working a double shift on Saturday, I am looking forward to a day of relaxation and personal time. But there is a problem. Sitting on the dining table in front of my breakfast is an assignment for a six-page U.S. History paper, which is due on Monday. Although I would prefer not to have to do the assignment, it is relatively painless. U.S. History is a subject I like and am good at. This essay should be a piece of cake for me.

My dilemma is that there is a football game today. The Patriots play the Jets at one o'clock. I am confident that I will easily write my paper, but the research and writing will occupy a large part of my day. I know that in the past things like this have been difficult for me to focus on for long periods of time. I decide to create a schedule. Over the past few months, my parents and teachers have tried to impress on me the value of creating and adhering to time tables in order to help me work on pace and finish on time. I decide, from considering a number of factors (familiarity with the subject, past performance, availability of research information), that this paper will take me 6 hours, start to finish. I allot 2 hours for researching the topic. The remaining 4 hours are for the actual writing. Normally I would allow for 1 hour of writing per page, but since I like history and because the last 2 pages will be opinion-based writing, I decide 4 hours is feasible. But then I get clever with my plan. I know that I am prone to distraction for assignments like this. So instead of the above pace, which assumes I am focusing fully on the task at hand, I double the time allotted for the writing portion of the assignment. By giving myself 8 hours to do a task that I am capable of doing in 4, I've successfully anticipated and dealt with my problems before they even arise. Now I've created a plan to follow and am more likely to be successful in writing my paper, and am also using a teacher- and parent-suggested technique for dealing with my focus problems. Satisfied and optimistic, I sit down in front of the TV with my laptop at 10 A.M., confident that by 8 P.M. I will be closing the laptop, having achieved both of my goals: a relaxing, stress-free day and a completed paper.

I work for 3 hours, finishing my research and getting through the introduction. So far I am on pace and have achieved my goal of working both casually and uninterrupted. My father comes into the living room at 1 to watch the opening of the game and check my progress. He knows about the paper, but I don't tell him about my schedule, just that I have everything under control. It is my plan, after all, and I am afraid that if I tell him about it he will criticize it before it even has a chance to work.

I watch the Patriots game and fall behind my pace, but with the padding I have given myself I have more than ample time to catch up. The four o'clock football game starts and I linger on it, thinking intermittently about how to begin my third paragraph.

My father returns, and when he sees how little progress I have made he gets agitated. We argue, me telling him that I have a plan and that how I choose to spend my time is my business. He says that I am putting my free time before my work and that mixing the two is counterproductive. He says that this isn't what he or the teachers had in mind—this isn't the plan they wanted. We yell and he finally leaves, saying that I am foolish for trying to have my cake and eat it too.

I finish the paper at 11 at night, writing the last three pages in an hour, after my dad came in and ordered me to shut the TV off. He told me that he knew this plan wouldn't work and that next time I should just do the work. Maybe he is right, but I won't admit it openly. In fact I insist that he distracted me from my work by criticizing my efforts to address my own problems. I tell him that he is being counterproductive by not allowing me to experiment with different methods for dealing with my responsibilities. He tells me that if he didn't put his foot down, I'd never get any work done.

(This is Dick talking:) This vignette, written by my son, Colin, depicts a situation that played out dozens of times between us when he was in high school. At the time, I saw his behavior as just one more example of context-dependent and task-avoidant behavior. Since I was focused only on the outcome (the paper), it took a long time for me to realize that I had missed an opportunity to help him develop and use his own problem-solving skills. Perhaps Colin would have finished the paper. If not, it might have been an opportunity for us to discuss his plan and make changes.

For parents of teens with executive skills weaknesses, when to risk short-term failure for a longer-term gain is an ongoing dilemma. The opportunity to fail is critical to learning, and parents need to be able to assess the potential costs versus the benefits of giving their teen the opportunity to fail. We are not advocates of a full-blown "tough-love" approach that says that teens will always learn from their mistakes. For adolescents with significant executive skills weaknesses, the proverbial "throw them off the dock to teach them how to swim" is likely to result in a string of failures, some of which may be catastrophic.

Instead, the goal of parents is to "keep them in the game" by providing enough frontal lobe support to help them evade major failures while at the same time giving them the chance to take risks and experience the consequences. We will provide guidelines for parents to assess risk versus reward—when it makes sense to give the teen some leeway and when it is time for the parent to step in and make a decision. Adolescents, fortunately, are somewhat ambivalent about their independence. While there are times when they resent their dependence and the meddling of their parents in their lives, there are other times when they seek out their parents for advice and support.

Our goal in writing this book is threefold: First, we want to help you understand what executive skills are and how these skills are the foundation for your teen's ability to live independently. Second, we want to provide tools to help you evaluate your teenager's specific executive skills as a way to understand where the teen may need support. And third, we want to provide specific and concrete information about how you can continue to act as "surrogate frontal lobes" for your teenager while at the same time respecting and fostering your teen's desire for independence.

We see adolescence as a time of great opportunity for parents. As we have noted, the brain is primed to acquire new abilities, and learning and practicing executive skills is key among these. Because of your changing relationship with your child during adolescence, you also have a unique opportunity to partner with your teenager in a way that provides guidance and at the same time provides direction for independence.

Why Does Your Teen Have Executive Skills Weaknesses?

There are at least three different sources of executive skills weaknesses in teens. The first is conditions or diagnoses characterized by deficits in executive skills. These include attention-deficit/hyperactivity disorder (ADHD), autism spectrum disorders, and traumatic brain injuries. The second source involves situations or conditions that are related indirectly to executive skills weaknesses. These include sleep disorders, mood disorders such as depression and anxiety, and habit disorders such as drug or alcohol abuse. The third source has to do with normal variations in executive skills.

Let's take the diagnoses first. Russell Barkley has made a compelling case that ADHD is first and foremost a disorder characterized by weaknesses in executive skills. Subsequent work by a number of researchers and clinicians in the field has added to the strength of this theory and helped to identify the executive skills typically affected. These routinely include response inhibition, attention, time management, planning and organization, and working memory and often involve the others we have discussed. The prototype for the "scattered teen" is the one who has ADHD. Since even conservative estimates conclude that 3 to 5% of the childhood population has ADHD, scattered teens exist in significant numbers.

Children on the autism spectrum, including those with Asperger syndrome, are also identified as having executive skills weaknesses. In our experience, problems with flexibility and emotional control are typical, as is difficulty with metacognition in the sense of being able to self-monitor and adjust behavior to the demands of a situation, particularly a social situation. Parents and teachers also report a range of other executive skills deficits.

In the case of traumatic brain injury, including multiple concussion injuries, impairments in executive skills are well documented and fairly common as a result of the susceptibility of the frontal lobes to acceleration/deceleration injuries where the head rapidly snaps back and forth. Weaknesses often include difficulty with response inhibition, flexibility, planning, working memory and, in teens, emotional control.

This doesn't cover all the populations for whom there is evidence of deficits in executive skills but does indicate some of the more common disorders associated with these weaknesses.

We recognize conditions indirectly related to executive skills deficits because these can be fairly common in adolescence. As we have noted, sleep deprivation adversely affects executive skills, and teens routinely suffer from sleep deprivation. Certainly we can see the impact of this on their attention or moodiness. As we also have seen, changes in the teen brain contribute to emotional highs and lows, including anxiety and depression, both of which can negatively impact executive skills. Changes in executive skills, among other behaviors, can also signal use of drugs or alcohol. In each of these circumstances, it is more recent or sudden changes that should lead parents to consider one of these causes.

We also recognize that executive skills weaknesses occur in the absence of a recognized disorder, diagnosis, or condition. Strengths and weaknesses are common among us. Do you know a person who is routinely late and seems to lack a sense of time urgency? How about the acquaintance who is disorganized and can't find belongings? Do you know someone who routinely "opens mouth, inserts foot"? These and other examples are quite familiar to us. In and of themselves, these weaknesses are no big deal unless they interfere with our ability to successfully negotiate problem situations, task demands, and social interactions.

It is for the population of teens whose executive skills weaknesses (regardless of their origin) interfere with successful problem solving and independent living that we have written this book.

2

Identifying Your Teen's Executive Skill Strengths and Weaknesses

Marco is a junior in high school. He's president of the student council and on the school's debate team. In these capacities, he can think on his feet and manufacture arguments out of thin air. When his proposal for a council project is met with resistance by the school administration, he can address objections and forge a compromise that gets the students what they want and satisfies the concerns of the principal. But take a look at his bedroom! Old candy wrappers litter the floor, the clean laundry is mixed in with the dirty, and his desk is piled high with a mix of school papers and notebooks, paperwork from clubs, and college guides (yes, he's already thinking about which colleges he might want to attend). Getting ready for school in the morning is inevitably a race against time as he tracks down the clothes he wants to wear and stuffs his homework hastily into his backpack—if he can find it. His teachers like him, and they sometimes give him a break when he persuades them that his homework is sitting on his desk at home and can he please, please, please bring it in tomorrow with no loss of credit, but Marco also recognizes that his report grades too often fall below his own goals because of his organizational problems.

Randy would seem to be a model student. A sophomore in high school, she's made the honor roll ever since sixth grade. She never hands in an assignment late, writes down clear directions in her agenda book, asks clarifying questions when she's not sure of what a project requires or what she needs to study for a test. Teachers love her (although some find her a little intense). "A little intense" doesn't begin to describe how she comes off at home, though. There her parents see her as a "bundle of nerves." She always seems to be in a panic about something—whether she has time to finish her art project, the topic she's going to write about for her World Cultures term paper, the B– she got on her last geometry exam, which threatens her A average. When her mom asks her to help out with the house cleaning on Saturday, she all but screeches at her: "I can't!! Do you know how much work I have to do?! You're totally messing up my life!" More often than not, her mom retreats. But she knows that the way Randy manages her emotions cannot be good for her, and she really knows it's affecting family life in a big—and bad—way.

If you absorbed the information in Chapter 1, you can probably do an informal assessment of the executive skills strengths and weaknesses of Marco and Randy. Both of them have some powerful strengths that contribute to their success as students and can predict positive outcomes as adults. They also struggle with some executive skills weaknesses that threaten to derail them. What they have in common is that their executive skills challenges are far more evident to their parents than they are to their teachers or other adults they come in contact with outside the home.

This makes parents uniquely able to identify and understand both the factors contributing to teens' success and the factors that may stand in the way of their ability to realize their hopes and dreams. Chances are you picked up this book because you are particularly focused on the latter. But in mapping out strategies to help your child cope with executive skills challenges, you need to start by getting a more complete picture of not just the teen's weaknesses but also the teen's strengths.

Why? For a number of reasons. First of all, so you can find something positive to celebrate in your child. The laser focus we often apply to problems and weaknesses sometimes leads us to overlook all the positives in our kids. Experts in a field called *positive psychology* have done extensive research documenting how effective positive feedback is on behavior, attitude, mood, and emotions. In fact, this research shows that receiving three pieces of positive feedback for each piece of negative or corrective feedback can produce positive behavior change all by itself.

Second, a complete picture will help you identify which areas of daily functioning you need to be most concerned about. For example, if your teen has

Executive Skills Required for Common Tasks of Daily Living for Teenagers

Executive skill	School performance	Completing college applications	Handling a busy schedule	Money management
Response inhibition				X
Working memory	X			
Emotional control			X	
Flexibility				
Sustained attention	X	X		
Task initiation	X	X		
Planning		X	X	
Organization		X		
Time management	X		X	
Goal-directed persistence	X	X		X
Metacognition	X			

Executive skill	Driving	Finding a job	Holding a job	Not engaging in risky behavior
Response inhibition	X		X	X
Working memory				
Emotional control			X	
Flexibility			X	
Sustained attention	X			
Task initiation		X		
Planning		X	X	
Organization				
Time management			X	
Goal-directed persistence		X		X
Metacognition				

weaknesses in task initiation and goal-directed persistence, school performance is likely to be a struggle. On the other hand, if sustained attention and impulse control are problems, driving will be a concern. The table on the previous page lists some common tasks we expect teenagers to perform along with the executive skills that are essential for performing those tasks successfully.

The sooner you can get a handle on your teen's executive skill profiles, the more likely you are to be able to intervene to help your teen improve his skills or develop effective compensating strategies. Teens vary in their willingness to accept suggestions from their parents, but the older they get the more likely you are to run into the teenage version of the 2-year-old's insistence that "I do it myself."

The executive skills questionnaires on pages 40–41 and 42–43 will help you and your teen assess her executive skills weaknesses. Complete the first one and then have your teen complete the second. Feel free to photocopy the forms if you want to use them more than once (such as for another teen or to have the teen's other parent complete the form).

What to Do with the Results

Start by comparing your estimates of your teen's executive skills strengths and weaknesses (the two to three lowest and highest scores) with your teen's estimates. The actual scores are less important than the listings of strengths and weaknesses. If they are very close, then you and your teen share similar perceptions of strengths and weaknesses. You might want to spend a few minutes talking about both the strengths and the weaknesses, beginning with the strengths. Share with your teenager how you see him drawing on his strengths in everyday life. Be specific in coming up with examples of how you've seen him use those strengths to manage task demands, solve problems, or handle sticky situations. Don't skimp on recognizing his strengths (remember: three positives for every corrective/negative!). If your child has a strength that is one of your weaknesses (more about that in the next chapter), it wouldn't hurt to say something like "I really admire the way you can . . . [accept constructive criticism, not put things off to the last minute, keep your desktop organized, etc.]. I wish I could do that better."

Next talk about the areas of weakness. Here, take your cues from your teenager. Have your daughter identify a weakness and talk about how it affects her ability to do something that's important to her. You might talk about how it's

Executive Skills Questionnaire—Parent Version

Rate each item below based on how well it describes your teen, using this rating scale to choose the appropriate score. Then add the three scores in each section. Use the key on the next page to determine your teen's executive skills strengths (two to three lowest scores) and weaknesses (two to three highest scores).

1	2	3	4	5	6	7
Strongly disagree	Disagree	Tend to disagree	Neutral	Tend to agree	Agree	Strongly agree

Item	Score
1. Acts on impulse.	____
2. Gets in trouble for talking too much in class.	____
3. Says things without thinking.	____
TOTAL SCORE:	____
4. Says "I'll do it later" and then forgets about it.	____
5. Forgets homework assignments or forgets to bring home needed materials.	____
6. Loses or misplaces belongings such as coats, mittens, sports equipment, etc.	____
TOTAL SCORE:	____
7. Gets annoyed when homework is too hard or confusing or takes too long to finish.	____
8. Has a short fuse—easily frustrated.	____
9. Is easily upset when things don't go as planned.	____
TOTAL SCORE:	____
10. Has trouble thinking of a different solution to a problem if the first one doesn't work.	____
11. Resists changes in plans or routines.	____
12. Has problems with open-ended homework assignments (e.g., doesn't know what to write about when given a creative writing assignment).	____
TOTAL SCORE:	____
13. Has difficulty paying attention—easily distracted.	____
14. Runs out of steam before finishing homework or other tasks.	____
15. Has problems sticking with schoolwork or chores until they are done.	____
TOTAL SCORE:	____
16. Puts off homework or chores until the last minute.	____
17. Has difficulty setting aside fun activities to start homework.	____
18. Needs many reminders to start chores.	____
TOTAL SCORE:	____

(cont.)

19. Has trouble planning for big assignments (knowing what to do first, second, etc.). _____
20. Has difficulty setting priorities when he/she has a lot of things to do. _____
21. Becomes overwhelmed by long-term projects or big assignments. _____

TOTAL SCORE: _____

22. Has disorganized backpack and notebooks. _____
23. Leaves desk or workspace at home or school messy. _____
24. Has trouble keeping bedroom or locker tidy. _____

TOTAL SCORE: _____

25. Has a hard time estimating how long it takes to do something (such as homework). _____
26. Often doesn't finish homework at night; rushes to get it done in school before class. _____
27. Is slow getting ready for things (e.g., appointments, school, changing classes). _____

TOTAL SCORE: _____

28. Can't seem to save up money for a desired object—problems delaying gratification. _____
29. Doesn't see the value in earning good grades to achieve a long-term goal. _____
30. Seems to live in the present. _____

TOTAL SCORE: _____

31. Lacks effective study strategies. _____
32. Doesn't check work for mistakes even when the stakes are high. _____
33. Doesn't evaluate performance and change tactics to increase success. _____

TOTAL SCORE: _____

KEY					
Items	**Executive skill**	**Items**	**Executive skill**	**Items**	**Executive skill**
1-3	Response inhibition	13-15	Sustained attention	25-27	Time management
4-6	Working memory	16-18	Task initiation	28-30	Goal-directed
7-9	Emotional control	19-21	Planning/prioritizing		persistence
10-12	Flexibility	22-24	Organization	31-33	Metacognition

Your teen's executive skills strengths (lowest score)	Your teen's executive skills weaknesses (highest score)
_____	_____
_____	_____
_____	_____

Executive Skills Questionnaire—Teen Version

Rate each item below based on how well it describes you, using this rating scale to choose the appropriate score. Then add the three scores in each section. Use the key on the next page to determine your executive skills strengths (two to three lowest scores) and weaknesses (two to three highest scores).

1	2	3	4	5	6	7
Strongly disagree	Disagree	Tend to disagree	Neutral	Tend to agree	Agree	Strongly agree

Item	Score
1. I act on impulse.	____
2. I get in trouble for talking too much in class.	____
3. I say things without thinking.	____
TOTAL SCORE:	____
4. I say, "I'll do it later" and then forget about it.	____
5. I forget homework assignments or forget to take home needed materials.	____
6. I lose or misplace belongings such as coats, gloves, sports equipment, etc.	____
TOTAL SCORE:	____
7. I get annoyed when homework is too hard or confusing or takes too long to finish.	____
8. I have a short fuse—am easily frustrated.	____
9. I get upset when things don't go as planned.	____
TOTAL SCORE:	____
10. If the first solution to a problem doesn't work, I have trouble thinking of a different one.	____
11. I get upset when I have to change plans or routines.	____
12. I have problems with open-ended homework assignments (e.g., deciding what to write about when given a creative writing assignment).	____
TOTAL SCORE:	____
13. I have difficulty paying attention and am easily distracted.	____
14. I run out of steam before finishing homework or other tasks.	____
15. I have problems sticking with schoolwork or chores until they are done.	____
TOTAL SCORE:	____
16. I put off homework or chores until the last minute.	____
17. I have difficulty setting aside fun activities in order to start homework.	____
18. I need to be reminded to start chores or homework.	____
TOTAL SCORE:	____

(cont.)

19. I have trouble planning for big assignments (knowing what to do first, second, ____ etc.).
20. I have difficulty setting priorities when I have a lot of things to do. ____
21. I become overwhelmed by long-term projects or big assignments. ____

TOTAL SCORE: ____

22. My backpack and notebooks aren't organized. ____
23. My desk or workspace at home or school is a mess. ____
24. I have trouble keeping my bedroom or locker tidy. ____

TOTAL SCORE: ____

25. I have a hard time estimating how long it takes to do something (such as ____ homework).
26. I often don't finish homework at night and may rush to get it done in school ____ before class.
27. I need a lot of time to get ready for things (e.g., appointments, school, ____ changing classes).

TOTAL SCORE: ____

28. I can't seem to save up money for a desired object—problems delaying ____ gratification.
29. I don't see the point of earning good grades to achieve a long-term goal. ____
30. I prefer to live in the present. ____

TOTAL SCORE: ____

31. I don't have very effective study strategies. ____
32. I tend not to check my work for mistakes even when the stakes are high. ____
33. I don't evaluate my performance and change tactics to increase success. ____

TOTAL SCORE: ____

KEY					
Items	**Executive skill**	**Items**	**Executive skill**	**Items**	**Executive skill**
1-3	Response inhibition	13-15	Sustained attention	25-27	Time management
4-6	Working memory	16-18	Task initiation	28-30	Goal-directed
7-9	Emotional control	19-21	Planning/prioritizing		persistence
10-12	Flexibility	22-24	Organization	31-33	Metacognition

Your executive skills strengths (lowest score)	Your executive skills weaknesses (highest score)
_____	_____
_____	_____
_____	_____

helpful to get a full picture of what's going on. "Now I see why you're late getting places. Time management is really hard for you, isn't it?"

But what if you and your child disagree on the profile? What if your teen sees as a strength what you see as a weakness? The temptation will be for you to amass evidence for why your teen is mistaken and hurl it at him. "Give me a break," you might want to say when your son thinks working memory is a strength for him. "Once a week for the last month you've called and asked me to bring you a homework assignment you left on your desk!" We would caution against taking this approach because it is likely to make your teen defensive and prompt an argument rather than an honest appraisal. A better approach would be to make a neutral comment. "Hmm, that's interesting, you and I see you pretty differently, don't we?" You might suggest that that difference in perception may be a cause for some of your conflicts. "You see yourself as having a great working memory—that must be why you get so aggravated when I say something to you like 'Did you remember to put your homework in your backpack?'"

Even if you disagree on what executive skills may be involved, the next step is to begin to tackle the situations that are either a source of family conflict or the ones that you deem as undermining your child's chance of success in whatever endeavor she is undertaking. The approach you will take depends in part on how your child responds to the feedback you give her indicating that there's a problem that needs to be addressed. We have identified five common ways many teenagers respond to a parental suggestion that they have a problem that needs to be fixed.

- *"I know I have a problem, but I can't manage it. Can you take care of it for me?"* Youngsters who respond in this way want someone else to solve the problem for them. Sometimes, although not often, it's as blatant as "Can you do my homework for me?" The more likely variations on this approach might be:

  - "Can you read over my essay and correct my mistakes?"
  - "If you think my room is too messy, you clean it up."
  - "Can you call my teacher and explain that I have ADHD and shouldn't be penalized for forgetting stuff?"
  - "I know I promised I would mow the lawn, but I forgot that the soccer season begins this week and I have practice every day. Can you give me a pass on the lawn mowing?"
  - "I *am* high-strung and I get stressed out a lot. That's just who I am, so you'll need to learn to live with it."

This approach sometimes irritates parents and sometimes elicits sympathy. If it get kids what they want—someone else to take care of the problem—then chances are their executive skills development will be slowed. *Tom's job is to make himself a sandwich every day before school. But whenever he forgets, his mother makes it for him; it worries her that he will have to go without lunch. But as a result, Tom never learns any memory techniques or sets any personal alarms, and his mother's gentle reminders do no good because they aren't backed by any tangible consequence.*

• *"I know I have a problem, I'm open to working on it, and I'm willing to get help from someone [of my choosing] if necessary."* Teens with this attitude are more open than many to taking steps to address the problem. These are kids who probably responded quite honestly to the executive skills questionnaire, and they may even offer a rueful laugh when they see their profile. Just because they recognize the problem and are willing to work on it, however, does not mean that they are looking for help from their parents. Some of our best coaching clients fall into this category: they're willing to work with a third party and they're even willing to work fairly hard as long as they are compatible with the person chosen to work with them. Although it may be hard for parents to step back and let someone else take on the helping role, this is actually a sign of maturity on the part of their children. These kids know they have to stop relying on their parents in order to take steps toward independence. A coach, a friend, or a trusted teacher can assist them with that process. Kailey always forgets her soccer bag when she's leaving for school and lately has gotten angry when her parents remind her over and over. She and two friends from the team decide that every morning they will all text each other about remembering their stuff for practice. With three people on this single task, there is a much better chance that they will all remember, and without parental help. We've devoted Chapter 20 of this book to an explanation of coaching and how teens and parents can make use of it.

• *"I admit I'm having a problem. Can we work out a deal that if I take steps to handle it I get something as a reward?"* Kids who take this approach often irritate parents because parents see themselves as having to *buy* behavior that should be given freely—especially since they see the ultimate goal as serving kids' interests more than their own. *Why should I have to pay my kid for something he should be doing anyway?* As with the previous approach, however, this one can be eminently workable for parents. With this approach, there's a built-in goal (improvement in the problem at hand) and a clear path to the goal (some kind of incentive). What's left is the negotiation between parents and kids to hammer out the details. *Danny wants new skis this winter. His parents agree that they will buy him the skis on the condition that he makes good grades. After negotiating, they decide that Danny will earn a certain percentage of the money he needs for the skis (or a differently priced pair) if he achieves a 3.0 GPA without having D's in any classes. For every point higher, he can earn more toward his goal (or a better pair of skis than a 3.0 would get him).*

- *"I guess I'm having a problem, but I'd like to handle it myself."* This response is more challenging for parents. A teenager who says this often has a long history of attempting—and failing—to handle things himself. *Darryl overlooks many things; he forgets to lock his car, regularly overdraws his checking account, and rarely responds to missed calls or voicemails. His parents try to help, but he insists that he can fix the problems himself. His parents think that while Darryl likes imagining himself as an adult, he has skipped over the learning and work required to really be one.* Again, parents are tempted to run down a litany of situations in which their child promised to handle something on his own, only to fall short. While this might work in a court of law before an impartial judge, it's unlikely to have the desired effect with an obstinate teenager. The better approach is offering to help your son create a plan for handling the problem and building in mutually agreed-upon markers for success.

- *"I don't think I have a problem, but if I do, don't worry—I'll take care of it."* Of the five options, this is the most frustrating for parents. You can see the problem clearly, and with the wisdom that years of experience bring you can see the disastrous outcome on the horizon if your teen fails to see and address the problem. If you have the luxury of time, you can inform your teen of what you will be looking for as evidence that she has "taken care of it" and let her know that if the evidence doesn't support her point of view, the issue will be revisited. If time is short (for example, the end of the marking period is fast approaching and she has two long-term projects that aren't close to being finished), you may need to take more intrusive steps.

Chapter 4 will go into more detail about how you can handle each of these response patterns. For now, let's see if you and your teen can agree on what response style he or she typically uses. Fill out the form on the facing page and have your teen fill out the teen version. Feel free to photocopy the forms to make extra copies for additional teens or your teen's other parent.

Compare the results. Do you and your teen agree on what his typical response style is? If you and he have trouble completing this assessment in the abstract, apply it to a specific problem that you would like to see addressed.

Parent Assessment

Which of the following response patterns does your child typically use when confronted with a problem involving executive skills weaknesses? Check off only one.

"I know I have a problem, but I can't manage it. Can you take care of it for me?"	
"I know I have a problem, I'm open to working on it, and I'm willing to get help from someone [of my choosing] if necessary."	
"I admit I'm having a problem. Can we work out a deal that if I take steps to handle it I get something as a reward?"	
"I guess I'm having a problem, but I'd like to handle it myself."	
"I don't think I have a problem, but if I do, don't worry—I'll take care of it."	

From *Smart but Scattered Teens*. Copyright 2013 by The Guilford Press.

Teen Assessment

Which of the following response patterns do you typically use when confronted with a problem involving executive skills weaknesses? Check off only one.

"I know I have a problem, but I can't manage it. Can you take care of it for me?"	
"I know I have a problem, I'm open to working on it, and I'm willing to get help from someone [of my choosing] if necessary."	
"I admit I'm having a problem. Can we work out a deal that if I take steps to handle it I get something as a reward?"	
"I guess I'm having a problem, but I'd like to handle it myself."	
"I don't think I have a problem, but if I do, don't worry—I'll take care of it."	

From *Smart but Scattered Teens*. Copyright 2013 by The Guilford Press.

This could be posed as: *I think you routinely leave papers until the last minute. As a result you pull an all-nighter and don't have time to proofread, much less do a thorough editing to improve your work. Which response option do you want to apply to this situation?*

Subsequent chapters will detail intervention strategies designed to address a host of executive skills difficulties. Which options are worth trying with your child depends in part on how your son or daughter completes the assessment.

3

Assessing Your Own Executive Skills and Parenting Style

Frank is a 50-year-old director of sales for a sports equipment company. He has no trouble running staff meetings, making cold calls to potential customers, and designing new marketing strategies that enable his company to expand beyond its traditional base. But his 17-year-old son knows how to push his buttons so that in the privacy of his own home he behaves in ways that he knows would shock customers and coworkers alike if they saw him in action. He keeps telling himself Jake has an attention disorder and is not capable of the same intense focus and task persistence that he has, but when he gets home after a late day at the office and sees him attacking aliens on his Xbox with no thought of homework and no memory of the project he promised his dad he'd start as soon as he got home from school, any rational thinking Frank may be capable of evaporates. Open mouth, spew forth rant. "Chill out, Dad!" Jake exclaims, reluctantly laying down the game controls. "I don't know why you get so upset. I asked my teacher for an extension, and she gave me till Monday. And besides, it's not like I haven't done anything! I worked for about half an hour after school, just like I said I would, but then I realized I left the directions for the project in my locker at school, and I need that to do the next step." Frank groans and with great effort tries to control his emotions. "Do you have other homework you should be working on?" he asks between clenched teeth.

Gina is a harried mother of four who also works part time managing the books at her husband's small consulting firm. Her kids range in age from 12 to 20, and she feels like it would be easier to run a multinational *corporation than try to stay on top of her kids' busy lives. She spends most of her day in her car, and she finds she's always running late. Her cell phone rings constantly, and it's usually a child asking her how soon she'll get there or whether she can please bring the homework inadvertently left on a desk in the bedroom. Her 18-year-old daughter is in the process of applying to colleges, and she's no better than her mother at remembering everything she has to do. She almost missed the deadline for signing up for her SATs, she can't remember which teachers she's asked to write recommendations for her, and she thinks she might have misplaced the folder her guidance counselor gave her with a list of things she has to do. "Mom, I know I need your help, because this is too complicated and too stressful for me to man- age on my own!" her daughter says, on the point of tears one evening after spending too long looking for that folder. Gina is flattered that her daughter is looking to her for assistance and not fighting her every inch of the way as her older brother did, but she's not sure she has the skills to be of much use to her. And the sleepless nights as she frets about this aren't helping either.*

If we want to help our kids become independent adults with fully func- tioning frontal lobes, as we can tell from these scenarios, *their* executive skills strengths and weaknesses are only half the puzzle. The other half is our own executive skills profile and how this impacts our ability to offer support, encour- agement, and in some cases ultimatums without causing damage to them or to our relationships with them. In the scenarios above, Frank's weak emotional control leads to conflict on a fairly regular basis with a son who appears to have not only a different executive skills profile but also a different set of priorities for his life. And Gina's weak time management skills and poor working memory, which may not be all that different from her daughter's skill levels in these areas, is a source of frustration to both Gina and her daughter. Complicating matters for all is the fact that so-called hot cognition (see Chapter 1) tends to turn up the volume on teens' emotions and, in turn, parent–teen conflicts.

Now that you've had a chance to assess your teen's executive skills strengths and weaknesses, you may have a good feel for what your own profile is. But in case any questions linger, take the rating scale on pages 51–52. Feel free to make a copy if your teen has another parent who wants to fill out the form too.

What to Do with the Results

First, look at your executive skills strengths. Try to remember when those skills became so strong for you. Maybe they've always been there (people with

Executive Skills Questionnaire for Parents

Rate each item below based on how well it describes you, using the following rating scale to choose the appropriate score. Then add the three scores in each section. Use the key on the next page to determine your executive skills strengths (two to three highest scores) and weaknesses (two to three lowest scores).

1	2	3	4	5	6	7
Strongly agree	Agree	Tend to agree	Neutral	Tend to disagree	Disagree	Strongly disagree

Item	Score
1. I tend to jump to conclusions.	____
2. I don't think before I speak.	____
3. I take action without having all the facts.	____
TOTAL SCORE:	____
4. I don't have a good memory for facts, dates, and details.	____
5. I am not very good at remembering the things I have committed to do.	____
6. I frequently need reminders to complete tasks.	____
TOTAL SCORE:	____
7. My emotions often get in the way when performing on the job.	____
8. Little things affect me emotionally or distract me from the task at hand.	____
9. I have trouble deferring my personal feelings until after a task has been completed.	____
TOTAL SCORE:	____
10. I get rattled when unexpected events occur.	____
11. I don't easily adjust to changes in plans and priorities.	____
12. I don't consider myself flexible and adaptive to change.	____
TOTAL SCORE:	____
13. I don't find it easy to stay focused on my work.	____
14. Once I start an assignment, I have trouble working diligently until it's completed.	____
15. When interrupted, I find it difficult to get back and complete the job at hand.	____
TOTAL SCORE:	____
16. No matter what the task, I have trouble getting started right away.	____
17. Procrastination is often a problem for me.	____
18. I often leave tasks to the last minute.	____
TOTAL SCORE:	____

(cont.)

19. When I plan out my day, I have trouble identifying priorities and sticking to _____ them.

20. When I have a lot to do, I find it hard to focus on the most important things. _____

21. I typically don't break big tasks down into subtasks and timelines. _____

TOTAL SCORE: _____

22. I am not an organized person. _____

23. It is difficult for me to keep my work area neat and organized. _____

24. I am not good at maintaining systems for organizing my work. _____

TOTAL SCORE: _____

25. At the end of the day, I usually haven't finished what I set out to do. _____

26. I am not good at estimating how long it takes to do something. _____

27. I am not usually on time for appointments and activities. _____

TOTAL SCORE: _____

28. I don't think of myself as being driven to meet my goals. _____

29. I don't easily give up immediate pleasures to work on long-term goals. _____

30. I usually don't focus on setting goals and achieving high levels of performance. _____

TOTAL SCORE: _____

31. I don't routinely evaluate my performance and devise methods for personal _____ improvement.

32. It is hard for me to step back from a situation to make objective decisions. _____

33. I don't "read" situations well and struggle to adjust my behavior based on the _____ reactions of others.

TOTAL SCORE: _____

KEY					
Items	**Executive skill**	**Items**	**Executive skill**	**Items**	**Executive skill**
1-3	Response inhibition	13-15	Sustained attention	25-27	Time management
4-6	Working memory	16-18	Task initiation	28-30	Goal-directed
7-9	Emotional control	19-21	Planning/prioritizing		persistence
10-12	Flexibility	22-24	Organization	31-33	Metacognition

Your strongest skills (highest scores)   **Your weakest skills (lowest scores)**

_____   _____

_____   _____

_____   _____

strengths in organization routinely tell us that they've *always* been organized), or maybe you had to work at them over time. I, for instance (this is Peg talking), am quite strong in task initiation, and yet one of my most vivid recollections of high school is dreading Sunday nights because English papers were always due on Mondays and I never started them until the night before. If your strengths happen to be different from those of your child, we urge you not to panic—your teen's deficit may simply reflect one of the slower-developing skills.

Next look at your weaknesses. How do those weaknesses impact your daily life? Have you put yourself in a job that minimizes the demands on those skills? Have you found someone to whom you can delegate tasks that require those skills? To what extent have your weaknesses prevented you from doing or achieving what you want—or have you found ways to work around them, maybe by using other skills? We've found, for instance, that people who have strengths in goal-directed persistence and weaknesses in task initiation are able to use their skill at doggedly pursuing goals to override their tendency to procrastinate. Understand again, though, that whatever your weaknesses are and whatever you've done to compensate for them, the process took time. You may have been well into adulthood before you figured out how to accentuate your strengths and downplay your weaknesses, and you can anticipate that the process for your child will be equally drawn out. Again, we urge patience when you think about your child's executive skill challenges.

Now line up your profile against that of your teen. Do you share strengths and weaknesses, or are your profiles markedly different? We have found that in any relationship (husband/wife, parent/child, teacher/student), tension points often arise when the strengths of one member of the relationship match up against the weaknesses of the other. This seems to arise because the one with the strength can't really conceive why it's a weakness for the other one. Those people who are naturally organized, for instance—it feels effortless to them to keep their workspaces clean and clutter to a minimum. For those of us who are not naturally organized, however, chasing clutter is so challenging and aversive that we put it off as long as possible or decide it's really not important anyway, so what's the big fuss? If that's how your adolescent responds when you bug her about one of her executive skills weaknesses, you can bet that doing what you've asked her to do feels so tedious to her that she can barely stand it. That's why teens with weak organizational skills *hate* to pick up their bedroom, clean out old papers from their notebooks, or put away the clutter on their desks so they have a clean space on which to study. Or ask a kid with weak working memory to make a list of things he has to remember to take to school tomorrow, and he looks at you as if you had just handed him a pencil and asked him to stick it in his eye.

Here's an important idea to keep in mind: effort is wholly in the mind of the beholder. When we hold seminars to explain executive skills, we routinely ask the audience to think about effort in the context of chores. We ask them to rate the kinds of household chores they do on a scale of 1 to 10, with "easy" chores falling at the low end of the scale—these are chores that we readily do and may even enjoy doing. Effortful chores fall at the high end of the scale— these are chores that we *hate* doing (even though we know how to do them); we put them off as long as possible, we coerce (or even pay) someone else to do them for us, or maybe we come as close to never doing them as we possibly can. We ask members of the audience to give us examples of chores that fall at the 1-2-3 end of the scale and chores that fall at the 8-9-10 end of the scale. Lo and behold, we find that a 1-2-3 chore for one person (say, cooking or mowing the lawn) is an 8-9-10 chore for another. The chore remains the same: the subjective reaction to that chore varies dramatically from person to person.

When you ask your teen to use an executive skill that's a weakness for him, you are asking him to do something that falls in the 8–10 range. If the same task happens to draw on one of your executive skills strengths, it may be hard for you to empathize or sympathize with your child. Maybe you've learned from years of experience that doing your chores early in the day or at a set time really works for you. Doesn't it drive you crazy when your daughter puts off loading the dishwasher until she should have been in bed half an hour ago—and then only because you nagged her? It may be easier for you to understand what's going on with your teen if you think about how hard you have to work at tasks that depend on one of your executive skills weaknesses. At least that levels the playing field a little (although not completely, since you need to remember that executive skills take 25 years to develop, or longer in young people with attention disorders or other learning challenges).

When we listen to parents and teens talk as they sit in our offices, we're struck by how often parents want to impart hard-earned knowledge based on their years of experience. "When I got to college, I learned I really had to plan my time carefully so that I could meet deadlines. This would be a good thing for you to practice," they say. Or "I've learned that by creating a good organizational system, I can work much more efficiently because I waste much less time looking for things I've misplaced." Parents who say things like this (and we all have!) fail to recognize two things. They appear to be unaware that their kids are not looking to them for advice as they may have when they were younger. They also don't seem to realize that the learning process that led them to these great systems and strategies took many years (and brain maturation) for them to master, and there may be no shortcuts to the time and practice their own kids will need to acquire the same skills and strategies. In the meantime, kids roll their eyes, make exasperated sounds, or tell their parents to stop talking (politely or rudely).

The benefits of completing the questionnaires in this chapter and the previous one are that you and your child gain a common language to talk about strengths and weaknesses. Here are some statements a parent might make to a teenager that use this common language:

> You know time management is one of my strengths and not one of yours, so I'm getting a little nervous right now about whether you've built in enough time to finish writing your English paper. Can you reassure me about this?

> I know you have trouble controlling your emotions sometimes, particularly when you're feeling stressed. Is there some way we can have a conversation about how you're going to make up your missing math assignments that can reduce that stress rather than make it worse?

> I admit it—I'm a neat freak, and organization is not one of your strengths. I'm wondering if we can reach a compromise in terms of keeping your bedroom picked up.

The Impact of Parenting Style on Executive Skills Development

Understanding your own executive skills profile and how it may differ from your child's facilitates communication, but we have found that a number of parenting styles make it difficult for parents to help their kids work on executive skills improvement. At the risk of overgeneralizing, this is how we'd describe them; try to look at yourself objectively to see if you fit any of these profiles:

• *Overinvolved or micromanaging parents.* Some parents doubt (perhaps with good reason) that their kids can succeed without close supervision. This is a natural response from parents who have seen their kids struggle with the same limitations for years and without any apparent improvement. Parents fear that if they don't fully deploy their own frontal lobes in the service of their children, their kids will crash and burn. So they issue frequent reminders, help organize bedrooms, backpacks, and notebooks, and may go so far as to do some of their kids' work for them—polishing English papers, filling out job applications, contacting potential colleges, helping to write the college essay. The list goes on and on. And their kids both resent the intrusion and come to depend on it, creating a lose–lose situation. Executive skills develop through practice—but with micromanaging parents, the opportunities for practice are often kept to a minimum.

• *Parents who would like to help but lack follow-through.* Some parents have great ideas for how to help their kids, and they may even be good at systems design, but they can't keep the system going. We see this particularly with parents who create checklists or behavior plans that include incentives. They initiate the process, but it gets lost over time. They may make a deal with their son that video games are off limits until nightly homework is done, but before long, they find him on Xbox as soon as he gets home from school. We also see it when parents promise to perform some task as part of the plan, and then they forget or their own lives become so busy they can't keep up their end of the bargain. A parent may agree to check her teen's assignment book nightly to make sure it's up to date or check in with the teen periodically to track progress on long-term assignments, and then the parent forgets to do so. Often this happens when parents fail to take into account their own executive skills weaknesses (for example, promising to provide cues or reminders when their own working memory skills are not so strong). Parents who lack follow-through end up discouraging both themselves and their children, and executive skill development gets sidelined. Teens are likely to conclude that if it's not important enough for the parents to follow through, then it's not important for the teen either. At the same time, the teen may also feel hurt because she interprets the parents' behavior as meaning *she's* not important.

• *Parents who are reluctant or afraid to confront their kids.* Some parents invest a lot in making excuses for their kids. They may take to heart the understanding that executive skills develop slowly or emerge late when children have attention disorders, and they're reluctant to hold their kids accountable. They decide that their kids should be allowed to hand in homework late because they forgot about it or left it at home, or should be allowed to retake tests when they fail the first one. While these may be reasonable accommodations for kids with ADHD, the danger is that kids will take advantage of the leeway they've been given, and then the executive skills will fail to improve—or may even decline. Or they feel bad that their child is having a tough time in some other arena (for example, difficulty making friends, going through the parents' divorce, having a learning disability that makes school hard), and they don't want to add to the child's misery. They prefer to blame themselves or blame circumstances rather than imposing consequences. These parents often intervene on their child's behalf rather than asking the child to self-advocate. "I forgot to remind you about your English assignment—I'll contact your teacher and explain the problem and ask if you can hand it in late." When this happens, unfortunately, the larger lesson children learn is that if they mess up, someone will bail them out.

• *Tough-love parents who feel that their children need to learn from unpleasant consequences.* It's true that children learn from mistakes, and we can't deprive them of that opportunity. But for youngsters with significant executive skills weaknesses, setting them up to fail repeatedly is not the answer. Tough-love parents often assume that the problems their child has can be chalked up to a motivational deficit: *If he cared, he'd keep his notebooks organized, he wouldn't lose his math homework, he'd plan his time better, he'd remember to hand in his chemistry labs on time. . . .* While motivation plays a role, we shouldn't discard the possibility that the child is hampered by a *skill* deficit: she really doesn't know how to keep her backpack organized or how to manage her time or to remember everything she has to do. In this case, punishment doesn't lead to improvement; it leads to continued failure, now with an emotional overlay that makes the matter worse. And that emotional overlay often plays itself out in increased tension and conflict with parents. Teens with parents like this often end up thinking there's nothing they can do to make their parents happy, so why even try.

• *Permissive/punitive parents who boomerang between expecting too much, imposing harsh consequences, and then letting everything slide.* These parents often begin as laissez-faire parents. They hope that their kids have their act together (these are "no news is good news" parents), and then when they find out they don't, they fly off the handle and, in a fit of pique, issue a punishment that is too harsh or unenforceable ("You're grounded for the rest of the marking period!"). With teens, taking away cell phones or car keys or access to electronics is often the penalty parents try to impose, but they go overboard and then allow their kids to whine and wheedle their way back to the privileges they were (briefly) denied. Their kids learn that if they wait, their parents will either forget the punishment or forget to impose it—or feel bad for losing their temper and retract it. The lesson kids learn with these kinds of parents is to hunker down and absorb the initial assault and then wait it out because it'll all go away soon.

• *Parents who disagree over how to handle the problem.* Sometimes in two-parent families, each parent has a different idea for how to handle their teen's executive skills weaknesses. When parents send mixed messages, the focus shifts away from executive skills development to the mixed messages themselves. When parents argue, disagree, or countermand each other, what the teen learns is that what's going on between parents takes precedence over his or her needs. Sometimes the teen is relieved ("Good—my parents are fighting and both have forgotten that I really screwed up"), but often the child feels confused and neglected ("I'm way less important to my parents than they are to each other"). If kids are looking for help, they're not getting it. If they're looking to avoid the problem altogether, parental disagreement may feed nicely into this—but the ultimate effect is that the child is not learning the skills needed for independence.

As Leo Tolstoy said, "Happy families are all alike; every unhappy family is unhappy in its own way." While there are a number of distinct parenting styles that can have a negative impact on executive skills development, effective parents—let's call them **authoritative/democratic parents**—generally use common methods. These are listed in the box below.

So what kind of parent are you—and would your teenager agree with your assessment? Parents and children often look at each other's behavior differently. Coming to some common understanding of what parenting style predominates can help you and your teen use the strategies in this book effectively. On the facing page you will find two quick rating scales—one for you to complete about

---

Authoritative/Democratic Parenting

To support executive skills development, *effective parents*:

- Solicit input from their teens and listen carefully to what they have to say.

- Are willing to give their teens a shot at solving the problem first before suggesting a solution.

- Use a collaborative approach to problem solving, working in *partnership* with their teens.

- Use communication techniques that convey respect.

- Share ideas and observations without being judgmental.

- Are willing and able to impose reasonable consequences when a deal has been made.

For Parents: What's My Parenting Style?

Read the descriptions and decide which style best reflects the one you use *most of the time*. If you feel you fluctuate between different approaches, select more than one (but no more than three!) and rank-order them, with 1 representing the style you use the most and 3 the least.

Parenting style	Ranking (1-3)
Overinvolved, micromanaging	
Would like to help, but follow-through is inconsistent	
Avoid confrontations at all costs (I know I need to hold my teen accountable, but I can't bring myself to do it)	
Tough love (children need to learn from their mistakes)	
Parents boomerang between overly permissive and punitive	
Parents disagree with each other about how to manage problems	
Authoritative/democratic—involving the teen in decision making and problem solving but also imposing rules and consequences	

For Teens: What Parenting Style Do My Parents Use?

Read the descriptions and decide which style best reflects the one you think your parents use *most of the time*. If you feel they fluctuate between different approaches, then select more than one (but no more than three!) and rank-order them, with 1 representing the style you use the most and 3 the least.

Parenting style	Ranking (1-3)
Overinvolved, micromanaging	
Would like to help, but follow-through is inconsistent	
Avoid confrontations at all costs (I get away with a lot because they don't have or enforce rules)	
Tough love (children need to learn from their mistakes)	
Parents boomerang between overly permissive and punitive	
Parents disagree with each other about how to manage problems	
Authoritative/democratic—they involve me in decision making and problem solving but also impose rules and consequences	

yourself and one for your teen to complete about you. These should be done separately, with no attempt by either party to influence the outcome. After you've each completed the survey, compare the results. Feel free to photocopy for another parent or if you have another teen you're concerned about.

How to Use This Information

First of all, look to see whether you and your teenager agree on your primary parenting styles. If so, then no matter what the style at least you can say you're all on the same page to begin with. If you and your son or daughter have radically different notions of how you parent, then the next step is to have a conversation so that you can understand your teen's point of view. Chances are your teenager can give you some good examples to support his or her perception. Listen and accept what the teen has to say. Then provide support for your point of view and ask if your teen can see where you're coming from.

Here's what that dialogue might look like:

"Mom, you say you see yourself as an authoritative/democratic authority type. Authoritative, sure, but I would say living with you is less a democracy and more a dictatorship. Remember a year ago when I wanted to go on that camping trip? You said no without getting any of the details, then grounded me for arguing, even though Dad said you guys would consider it."

"Fair enough, Kerry. I'll admit that there have been times when I was less than flexible. But you can be very combative when it comes to getting your way; sometimes I react strongly because I think there is a fight coming, that you'll lash out at me regardless of how I say no."

The goal is to move toward an authoritative/democratic approach, so the next step is to talk about how that might be achieved. You might say something like this:

I realize I've made some mistakes and misjudgments along the way. [Summarize what these are, which will depend on your predominant parenting style—I haven't given you a chance to prove yourself because I've been on top of you all the time; I haven't followed through with what I've promised to do for you; I've been afraid to impose consequences because I didn't want you to hate me; I haven't imposed consequences because I felt bad about some of the burdens you have to deal with; I've gone too far in assuming that you need to learn from your mistakes and haven't given you the support you need to succeed; I've let things slide, hoped for the best, and then blown up when I was disappointed; Your dad and I have disagreed on how to handle things and sent you mixed messages.]

I want to try to do better because I think you need support and consistency, and I need to listen more and involve you in the problem solving and decision making. The whole point of this is to help you learn to make good decisions, so your input will be important. At the same time, I need to keep doing my job as a parent, and that means that if I see problems with doing things *your way,* there will be times I need to override your preferences. Parenting is an art, when all is said and done, and if you and I disagree about things, I will need to decide whether this is a situation where, if we do it your way and it doesn't work out, no serious harm will be done and you might learn something valuable *or* whether this is something where the stakes are just too high and I can't take that risk. I wonder if we can agree that I will consider your input and whenever possible incorporate your ideas and suggestions, but that if the ultimate decision goes against what you want, you will recognize that the decision I'm proposing comes from my love for you and from my genuine desire to have you avoid making a mistake that will prove too costly.

If you would like to be able to have this kind of conversation with your teen but feel that the relationship is too difficult or hostile to be able to pull it off successfully, you may want to enlist the services of a third-party mediator to help you have this discussion. If your relationship with your teen is not troubled by significant conflict, a wise family friend might do the trick. If the issue centers on academics, a coach (see Chapter 20) might be a good choice. Otherwise a counselor or therapist is probably best.

If you can have this discussion and you feel it goes well, you're probably ready to consider the suggestions provided in the rest of this book. We will try to lay out different options depending on the degree of cooperation you can count on from your teenager, but the more you and your child can agree on key issues—such as both of your executive skills strengths and weaknesses, your child's style of responding to your suggestions, and the parenting style that you're shooting for—the more likely it is that the ideas we have to offer will be workable.

Part II

LAYING A FOUNDATION
THAT CAN HELP

4

....

Ten Principles for Improving Your Teen's Executive Skills

Now we're about to get into the nuts and bolts of helping your teen improve his or her executive skills. You've learned what executive skills are, how they manifest themselves in day-to-day situations, and how they develop over time. You understand the role of brain systems in executive skills, the developing but incomplete state of teen brains, and the opportunities and challenges this presents for parents. Chapter 2 has given you the tools to gather some key pieces of information that can guide your efforts: how you view your child's strengths and weaknesses, how your child views them, whether your assessments agree, and how your teen is likely to respond to feedback from you when there is a problem. This information about your child's skills represents one half of what you need to know before the two of you can work together. In Chapter 3 we've given you the tools to get the other half—what your executive skills strengths and weaknesses are and the type of approach that most often represents your parenting style.

Out of this information, different scenarios can arise. Suppose, for example, that one of your strengths is one of your child's weaknesses. You may find it hard to believe that your teen doesn't have this skill because you easily solve problems that require the skill. Or if you have a "tough love" parenting style, your child's missteps may seem like a motivational issue that will be resolved by letting the teen just suffer the consequences. Sometimes parents assume that children will acquire executive skills through their daily living experiences at home and in school, or they are reassured by teachers that learning these skills is a natural part of adolescent development.

Perhaps your parenting style is one of micromanagement, and until now you've been an effective "surrogate frontal lobe" for your child. Now, however, you're getting some pushback from him, and you are wondering if there's a way to step back without seeing him flounder.

Maybe your child has repeatedly insisted that she could handle a problem on her own and you've seen a series of unsuccessful attempts. Now you're searching for a way to help her while at the same time letting her save face and move toward self-management.

Up to the present, maybe your teen has done well with you providing reminders and creating organizational schemes. However, looking down the road you can see that he will be moving on and therefore needs to develop his own self-cuing strategy.

Perhaps your teen is open to help from you and you're unsure how much help to provide or when to pull back. You don't want her to become dependent on you, but you also don't want her to fail.

Or you might be facing the opposite scenario, where your teen has dug in and refuses to acknowledge that there is any problem, but you feel that if you don't push your child to act, your inaction could result in problems from which she can't recover.

In this chapter, we have set out 10 principles to guide you in helping your teen. You can use them to develop strategies that take into account your teen's unique circumstances and characteristics. A number of them also serve as a guide to minimizing the inevitable divides and reducing the conflicts in parent–teen interactions. You will see several of these principles spelled out in much greater detail when we begin talking about interventions in the following chapters.

1. Don't assume that a struggling teen has executive skills and is not using them.

Once children reach adolescence, we adults tend to see their use of executive skills as a matter of motivation: "Of course Jason should be able to resist his friends' pressure to drink. He just doesn't want to be left out." "Emily knows very well how to keep her assignments organized. She just gets lazy about keeping her binders up to date." The problem with this attitude is twofold: that the teen has the requisite executive skills and that the teen isn't motivated to use them are *both* questionable assumptions. Maybe it's the fact that we've seen them grow so much in so many different ways that makes us believe our teenagers have the skills they need to succeed. After all, they've been taught, they've had plenty of chances to practice, they've had the skills modeled for them, and they've seen what happens when kids exhibit poor impulse control and let chaos reign in their schoolwork and elsewhere. They *must* know how to inhibit impulses and how to stay organized, among other skills. But do they really? What did the questionnaires in Chapter 2 reveal about your teen's executive skills strengths and weaknesses? And think about it for a minute: Sure, adolescents can be lazy (or is it exhausted and distracted?), but if they really do have the skills to succeed and they really have seen what happens when someone yields to every impulse and is completely disorganized, why wouldn't they be motivated to use those skills?

While motivation can play a significant role in teens' behavior, it's important to recognize that some behaviors reflect a skill weakness rather than a lack of motivation. As we discussed in Chapter 3, and as you are probably aware from having assessed your own executive skills, we all have strengths and weaknesses. To evaluate weaknesses in your teen, be aware of his capacity to engage in effortful (and nonpreferred) mental tasks. If he is bright and a good "consumer" of information (interested in a range of topics, likes to read and watch educational programs), but is not a good "producer" of information (struggles with projects, papers, etc.), executive skills are likely involved. Here are some tips for knowing whether your teen has the skills and knows how to apply them:

- Looking back at when your son or daughter was younger, did teachers comment about any issues with organization, time management, finishing work, needing reminders to stay on task, and so forth?

- Were you a fairly regular visitor to the "lost and found" in elementary school?

- Have you seen examples of your teen's ability to perform at a high level and felt that if only she could sustain that level or find something that she was really interested in, she would "take off" and achieve the potential that you've seen at times?

- When your teenager reached middle school, did some teachers begin to question his motivation or even suggest that he was lazy? Did you hear more than once that "he needs to put in more effort" or "he isn't working up to his potential" or "he has good ideas but can't seem to get them down on paper"?

- As homework has increased, is procrastination or timely completion an ongoing problem, even though once your teen starts her homework, she can complete it without help? Have you thought or said to your teen more than once, "If you spent half as much time doing your homework as arguing about it, you'd be done already"?

- When your child got to middle school, did his grades decline from elementary school, even though they remained decent?

- Do you find yourself having to remind or "nag" your teen on a regular basis to watch the time, remember sports equipment, start or finish chores, get up in the morning?

- Does she routinely opt for the fun stuff in spite of having schoolwork to do?

- Do you find yourself regularly monitoring your teenager's TV watching, online social networking, texting, etc.?

- Does he have trouble following through even on activities that you know he is interested in?

If you see your teen in some of these descriptions and he or she continues to struggle, it's likely that one or more executive skills weaknesses are involved. Considering this information together with what you found out in the assessment in Chapter 2, from your perspective what skill or skills should be your top priority? To help your teen develop those skills, keep the following principles in mind.

Drew's parents often fought with him over his study habits; they said his frequent texting and dallying on the Internet was harming his grades. But when they restricted him from using these things while he was working, he still had difficulty focusing on his work. His parents realized that outside distractions weren't the only problem, but that Drew also had issues with attentiveness and goal-directed persistence.

2. You will need to help your teen learn these skills; your son or daughter won't acquire them through observation or osmosis.

Some teens have a natural capacity for observing and using executive skills effectively, while others stumble and struggle if left on their own. Many parents and teachers foster executive skills development through what psychologists call *incidental learning*—that is, they provide loose structures, models, and occasional prompts and cues, and that is all that's needed. Or perhaps it was all that was needed in simpler times, when the demands on teens were fewer and where the amount of supervision and support that parents and teachers could provide was greater. In this day and age, however, we are seeing an explosion in the amount of information available and the speed with which it is processed, thanks to communications technology available to teens. As a result, at one point or another most teens struggle with some task that requires a level of executive functioning that is beyond them.

To respond to this more complex world, we can't leave executive skills development to chance. However, working with teens on these skills is not like working with younger children. At this stage of their development, they are unlikely to tolerate our telling them, on a day in, day out basis, how to organize their belongings or manage their time or emotional reactions. Even if they tolerated this, it would not be in our interest or theirs to make all of their decisions for them, because to do so undermines their growth and development. At the same time, we recognize that we have to be part of this decision-making process because our teens are not yet sufficiently skilled to make decisions with complete independence. In attempting to find this balance between assistance and independence, the following principles are critical.

Emily's son Tom regularly misses appointments and is late for school, and simple reminders aren't helping. Emily sits down with Tom and explains her system of self-reminders, including her day planner and smartphone. She also talks to Tom about the importance of factoring in buffer time between activities to account for unexpected events. She initially sends the reminders to him via text and works with him until he reliably uses the reminder function on his own phone.

3. Understand your teen's innate drive for mastery and control and focus on opportunities for the teen to pursue objectives related to independence.

One of the fundamental and critical differences between working with your younger child on executive skills and working with your teenager is the teen's rapidly developing need for control and independence. This situation presents both significant opportunities and significant challenges for parents. The opportunity comes because your adolescent is seeking the same outcome for herself as you are. Namely, she wants to make decisions for herself and to be as independent as possible. Since independent living is the same outcome that parents want for their children, on the face of it, this time in the lives of a parent and adolescent could be an ideal situation. Unfortunately, at times it is not, especially for the parents of a teenager with weak executive skills. The reason for this is that parent and teen have fundamentally different points of view about the ability of the teen to make good or safe decisions. Teens typically don't question their ability to make decisions for themselves, at least in front of their parents. However, this confidence does not necessarily translate into good decision making. The challenge for parents is twofold: You have to hand off the decision making and problem solving to the teen in a way that promotes the development of good decision-making ability and at the same time recognize that some decisions need to remain in your hands. From the teenager's perspective, any shared or especially sole decision making by parents may be frustrating. This leaves you with the task of searching for opportunities to encourage the drive for mastery and control in your teen without putting her at significant risk. One way to do this is to work with your teen on accomplishing objectives that are in the teen's self-interest and that signify increased independence. For example, you could work together to help your teen obtain a driver's license or purchase a car. In Chapter 5, involving motivation, we'll expand on these types of examples as a way for you to work with your teen on executive skills in areas where the teen is motivated to succeed.

The Sanders family had to go to a relative's wedding in Vermont, and they needed to book a hotel. They asked their son Todd to find accommodations because he was planning a ski trip with friends and they wanted to give him a chance to practice finding affordable lodging.

4. While the long-term goal is to reduce support and promote independence, a key role for you is also to "keep your teen in the game."

You want experience to be a teacher, but you do not want your teen to commit catastrophic errors (failure in high school or early college, unsafe driving, drugs or alcohol, unsafe sex). To understand how to accomplish this, you have to have an accurate understanding of the type and magnitude of your teen's executive skills weaknesses. Weaknesses in some executive skills represent less risk than others. For example, while a weakness in working memory can negatively impact school performance, there are tools and strategies available to help (cell phones, school websites, etc.) that are not particularly intrusive and that can promote increased independence over time. A weakness in goal-directed persistence is more problematic since the teen does not readily connect what happens today with the distant future, which means you have to find a way to motivate your teen to do tasks that currently may seem meaningless or irrelevant until your son or daughter does develop more future orientation. Or, suppose your child's weakness is in attention. Given all the potential distractions that teens face (music, cell phones, peers) and their lack of experience, driving represents a major risk. While the easy solution—don't let your attention-challenged teen drive until he's older—might solve the problem for you, for the adolescent this solution threatens one of the most fundamental signs of independence and in a concrete way keeps the teen tied to home, a result that likely will lead to significant conflict. Similar but even more difficult decisions confront parents whose adolescent is weak in response inhibition. Driving, access to alcohol or drugs, and sexual relationships, especially in the context of peer influence, all represent genuine risk for the teen who tends to act before she thinks. Attempts to restrict or heavily control your teen's access to peers based on your fears of the consequences are also likely to lead to major conflicts.

But make no mistake about it, if your teen is to achieve adequate self-management and independence, you will have to be prepared to take some risks, and at times the risk will be significant. In negotiating this minefield, you'll have to continuously define and redefine what you consider acceptable risk. In Chapter 6, on environmental modifications, we will detail a number of alterations and interventions that you can introduce to at least decrease these risks.

Tina's grades kept slipping, but she insisted on managing things herself. She and her parents agreed that they wouldn't intervene, as long as Tina showed evidence (e-mails, etc.) that she had met with her teachers to establish a plan for her to get back on track, and her grades on PowerSchool (a school information portal that parents can access online in many school districts) reflected this.

5. Move from the external to the internal.

As we have mentioned, you acted largely as your child's frontal lobes when your son or daughter was really small. All executive skills training begins with something outside the child. Before your child learned not to run into the road, you stayed with him and held his hand when the two of you reached a street corner to make sure that didn't happen. Eventually, because you repeated the rule "Look both ways before crossing," your child internalized the rule, then you observed your child following the rule, and eventually he could handle crossing the street by himself. In all kinds of ways, while your child was growing up you organized and structured his environment to compensate for the executive skills he had not yet developed, and you will continue to do that now that your child has reached adolescence. At the same time, you realize that he will not accept the same type of handholding or direction from you that he accepted when he was younger, so the external changes that you make with your teenager are quite different but no less necessary.

Remember that the external includes changes you can make in the environment, the task, or the way you interact with your child. For the teen, environmental changes could range from something as simple as providing an alarm clock to as sophisticated as finding cars with extensive safety features and the capacity for driver monitoring. Changing a task might involve starting with smaller steps, since the teen has not consistently met the expectations for the larger task. For example, instead of room cleaning, putting dirty clothes in the laundry basket could be a first step. In terms of how you interact with your teen, communication strategies are key, and we will have much more to say about these in the following chapters.

When Jeff kept forgetting his backpack, his parents put a different-colored Post-it on the door every day, reminding him to take it. Gradually they shifted to every other day, and then to an alarm on Jeff's phone that rang while he was eating breakfast. Over time, Jeff learned to internally remember to take his backpack.

6. Work with your teen on strategies to assist her without annoying or alienating her.

This means understanding her style and strengths and focusing on communication, negotiation, and choice. To maintain a relationship with your teen, it's important to be aware of your teen's style or attitude, which we discussed in Chapter 2, as well as your own parenting style, addressed in Chapter 3. Understanding your teen's style determines in part how you will approach him. As we have noted, the teen who is open to negotiation is very different from the teen who sees all attempts to discuss problems or issues as "none of your business." If you tend to parent from a position of authority, your teen is likely to react very differently than if you parent from a position of negotiation and choice. Demands and ultimatums from parents leave little room for decision making by the teen and are likely to lead to increasing conflicts and defiance, as the teen sees this as a battle for control. Both you and your teen will benefit from your efforts, whenever possible, to engage in a discussion about expectations and rules. Your teen will also respond positively when you make an effort to help her recognize and play to her strengths. Comments such as "You did a nice job talking with your brother when he got into your stuff" or "I really appreciated your stopping at the store to pick up the vegetables for dinner" recognize behaviors related to executive skills and present the opportunity for you to build on these. As we noted in Chapter 3, understanding your own executive skills and the match or mismatch between your skills and your teen's will also help you deal with communication issues. Because it seems easy to you does not mean it's easy for your teen. Resist the urge to critique her efforts as inadequate and to offer your own as a better alternative, or to minimize the problem. You'll know you're in this territory if you hear yourself saying, "It's easy; all you have to do is . . . " Teens are also more likely to be open to suggestions and assistance from parents when they understand that their parents love them and offer assistance because they want them to be safe and to have choices and opportunities for themselves in the future. Although this may seem self-evident to you, it is not always evident to teens and bears repeating to them. We will discuss specific communication strategies as a key environmental modification in Chapter 6.

Kayla hates chores; she is easily distracted and can drag even simple tasks out for hours. But she loves running errands and is good at following even complex sets of directions. Therefore, her father eases her into chores in short, very finite time slots and regularly weaves them in with trips to the store for household items.

7. Consider your teen's developmental level and capacity to exert effort.

We don't expect 5-year-olds to plan and prepare the lunches they take to day care, and we don't expect 14-year-olds to live in their own apartment, yet in our clinical practice, parents hold unrealistic expectations for their teen's level of independence. For example, we routinely work with parents of high school freshmen or sophomores who are irritated because their kids do not yet have a clear idea what college they want to go to after they graduate or understand what they need to do to get into that college. It is not unusual, in our experience, for even high school seniors to need assistance with this process from parents, guidance counselors, or both.

Understanding what is normal or typical at any given age so that you don't expect too much from your teen is the first step in addressing executive skills weaknesses. We included a table in Chapter 2 that lists the types of tasks involving executive skills that it may be reasonable to expect a teen to perform. But knowing what is typical for most teens is only part of the process. When your own teen's skills are delayed, you need to step in and intervene at whatever level your child is functioning now. That is, you will need to match the task demands to your teen's actual developmental level, even if that is different from that of his peers or from what you would like it to be.

You also have to modify tasks to match your teen's capacity to exert effort. Some tasks require more effort than others. This is as true for adults as it is for teens. Think of that task at home that you keep putting off—you know, the one that makes you think of a million things you have to do that are more pressing. In fact, though, there are two kinds of effortful tasks: ones you're not very good at and ones you are very capable of doing but just don't like doing. The same is true for teens, and different strategies apply depending on which kind of task is under consideration.

If we're talking about tasks that the teen is not very good at, you handle them by breaking them down into small steps and starting with either the first step and proceeding forward or the last step and proceeding backward, and you don't proceed to the next step until the teen has mastered the previous step. Take laundry as an example. Beginning at the end would mean your doing the entire task except the last step (pulling the washing machine knob out and closing the top). Starting at the beginning might mean asking the teen simply to sort the clothes into light and dark. You praise the teen for doing a good job and move past that first step only when it becomes second nature. But really, it is the second kind of effortful task that parents tend to have strong feelings about. These are the ones where you might have accused your teen of "just deciding he doesn't like to do them." If the task has become a battleground between you and your teen, it has probably gone beyond a simple decision on the part of the teen that the task is distasteful. Our approach is: If you fought that battle a couple of times and didn't win, it is best to change the nature of the battle. Your goal is to teach the teen to exert effort by helping him override the desire to quit or do something else that is preferable. The way to do this is to make the first step so easy that it does not feel particularly hard to the teen and immediately follow that first step with some type of reward. The reward is there to ensure there is a payoff for the teen from expending the small amount of effort it takes to complete the first step. You then gradually increase the amount of effort the teen has to expend to achieve the reward.

Finally, don't assume that because the solution looks simple to you it's a simple solution. This is especially important if your strength is your teen's weakness. When you are strong in a particular executive skill, solutions to problems involving that skill will come easily. Let's take organization. Looking at your teen's living space may almost instantly trigger notions of how to organize the space. If organization is not your teen's strong suit, the same scheme will not be apparent to him. In addition, since he's a teenager, simply accepting and implementing your plan might threaten both his need for autonomy and his sense of confidence. Hence you may need to approach the situation from the perspective of helping someone learn the skill who has no idea where to begin, and to do that your teen must have some motivation for or see some payoff in the task.

Brenda was having trouble getting her daughter to complete the tasks she was asked to do. When confronted, her daughter confessed that some of the tasks, like making appointments or getting her car repaired, intimidated her. Brenda promised to help her daughter gain confidence in these areas by coaching her about what to say when she made the calls.

8. Provide just enough support for your teen to be successful.

This principle appears to be so simple as to be self-evident, but in fact implementing the principle may be trickier than it appears, especially for teens. The principle includes two components that are of equal weight: (1) *just enough support* and (2) *for the child to be successful*. Parents and other adults who work with teens tend to make two kinds of mistakes. They either provide too much support, which means that the teen is successful but fails to develop the ability to perform the task independently, or they provide too little support, so that the teen fails and, again, never develops the ability to perform the task independently.

For parents of teens, the first step in this principle is recognizing what you have done and may continue to do for your teen that the teen could, and perhaps should, begin doing on her own. Here we are thinking about activities such as laundry, setting up doctors' appointments, getting up in the morning, and managing money. In Chapter 7 we'll suggest specific plans for a variety of routines and activities that you might choose to begin working on with your teen. All of these involve skills that your teen will require to live independently as an adult.

For now, let's return to the two elements of the principle. In helping teens learn a skill by taking on new tasks, we assume that at the beginning stages the teen will need support. For a teen it's best to determine how far he can get in the task on his own and then intervene. You may be able to do this by simply asking him how to proceed through the task. In other cases, he may agree to take on the task, but then you notice that he hasn't made progress in moving through the task. If this occurs in activities where he is likely motivated, such as setting up a bank account, exploring the process for getting a driver's license, or getting a job, this may be a sign that in spite of what he said he is not sure how to get started.

Keep in mind that teens are inclined to either think or say that they can manage something, even when they are not sure. In this case, a gentle and even tentative offer of information or help may get a teen started and help her be more comfortable with enlisting your aid for additional steps. The second part of the principle, *for the teen to be successful*, is the real criterion for determining whether she has had enough support. If she's open to your help but you stepped back too early in the process, and as a result your teen doesn't successfully complete the activity, her confidence will be undermined. You want to think about this as being behind your teen and providing enough support so that she successfully crosses the finish line with you watching from the back, cheering her on, not in front, reaching the finish line first.

Michael and Karen always assumed that they would need to constantly look over their son Spence's shoulder for him to achieve his academic goals; they had been doing this since he was in first grade. But as teachers became less receptive to providing them with almost daily updates, and Spence himself complained that they were suffocating him, they realized that loosening the reins would be beneficial to everyone. Now Spence is the liaison between his parents and instructors, and his teachers contact Michael and Karen only when Spence misses a major assignment or his grade drops below a B.

9. Keep support in place until the teen achieves mastery or success.

We see parents who know how to help a teen break down tasks into manageable steps, teach or model the skills that will be needed, and reinforce successes along the way, and yet the teen still fails to acquire the skill. More often than not, this is because of a failure to apply this principle and/or the next one. These parents may help to set up a process or procedure, see that it is working, and then back out of the picture, expecting the teen to keep succeeding independently. Here it will be essential to understand your child's behavioral history. If over the course of your child's development you've had the experience of working with the child on an activity or skill, seeing progress, and assuming that the issue was taken care of, only to find out that over a period of days or weeks after you withdrew your support the child began to fail, then assume you will need to stay in the picture longer. This can be tricky with teens since they may either not want you in the picture to begin with or want you out of the picture as quickly as possible. If this is the case, then at the very least you can provide support by being an active observer and step in with an offer of help or support when you see that your teen has stopped moving forward or is beginning to slide back. Teens are much more likely to be open to offers of help or support if they feel that your offers come because you want what is best for them and that you will support them in their decisions even if their goals are not necessarily your goals.

Given this ongoing and delicate balancing act between teens and parents involving support versus independence, there is plenty of opportunity for disagreement and conflict. Expect your teen to push you away or even reject offers of help even if it seems that the teen is also searching for support. It's important not to become so annoyed with this confounding behavior that you simply walk away. At one time or another you've probably felt "Well, since he doesn't want my help, let's see what he can do on his own." You may have been thinking more along the lines of teaching your teen a lesson than paving his path to success. While you may prove your point in an "I told you so" kind of way, your relationship will inevitably suffer, and your teen is likely to be both discouraged and angry and less likely to listen to you in the future. Most important, he is no closer to independence and a sense of self-mastery. In spite of the conflict, the objective is not for you to play "gotcha" to demonstrate your teen's weakness, but to keep track of things and to offer assistance as needed for the teen to be successful.

Allie wanted to manage her own wake-up time with an alarm in the morning, but her mother routinely went to her room to make sure she was up because tardiness had been an issue when she was a freshman. They agreed that Mom would check only if she wasn't downstairs by 6:45. This happened only four times during the term, and when she did check, Allie was up and nearly ready. They agreed that Mom would drop the checks unless Allie wasn't up before Mom left the house at 7:10.

10. When you do stop the supports, fade them gradually, never abruptly.

Even if you stick with the supports that you put in place long enough to allow your teen to do the task or use the skill independently, at that point you may be tempted to assume that the issue is resolved and stop the support. Instead, you need to fade the supports gradually so that the teen can continue to demonstrate and extend independence with this skill. Let's think about the bike-riding analogy. If you've ever taught a child to ride a bike, you know that you start by holding on to the back of the bike and keeping it upright, and every once in a while, as your child practices, you let go for a second or two to test whether the child can keep the bike going without too much wobbling. If so, you gradually let go for longer and longer. You don't hold on to the bike constantly and then suddenly just "let her fly" and expect the child and the bike to keep going without a crash. And even when the child does ride independently, you maintain support for a time by limiting where and when she rides and watching her, ever available to come to her assistance if she does crash, helping her get back on her feet, and encouraging her to continue, putting the fall in the category of minor and accepted setbacks that are part of the learning process. We want to provide the same gradual fading of support and encouragement to continue whether it involves turning the whites in the laundry pink because of errant sorting or encouraging a teen to drive again after an accident because of errant attention.

Asima and her parents have a deal: the computer and cell phone are off limits until her schoolwork is done, and she leaves them in the kitchen while doing homework. When her progress report comes back strong, her parents are ecstatic and lift the ban on mixing homework and electronics. Within 2 weeks, Asima is behind on her assignments and is distraught. She and her parents sit down and agree that they will remind her not to use them and will monitor intermittently. Asima commits voluntarily to avoiding these distractions. When her next report is positive, they agree to let her try mixing homework time and electronics, and they check her completion of assignments through the parent portal on PowerSchool once or twice a week.

You should be able to rely on these principles whenever you are deciding how to approach a problem with your teen or whenever you want to help your daughter or son hone an overall skill. In fact, you might find it helpful to review these principles anytime you find yourself stalled while using the strategies in Chapters 9–19. Sometimes we forget how important it is to stick to the ground rules when life and its demands—on us and our kids—get complicated.

5

....

Motivating Your Teen
to Use Executive Skills

You've undoubtedly heard the following words, or some variation of them, since your teen was 3 or 4 years old, or maybe even younger:

"No!"

"I do it myself!"

"You're not the boss of me!"

These statements are typically accompanied by behaviors that signal the child's budding desire for self-management and decision making, independent of what you want. Frustration with the behavior aside, you can smile at the child's attempt to take control of her life, although she has no idea what that really means other than for this moment. At the same time, when our children make these statements, it is a testament to how powerful the drive for autonomy is and a sign of developments to come.

During adolescence, "I do it myself!" takes on a whole new meaning and requires parents to recognize two facts. The first is that in the next few years, for most adolescents, this will become a true statement. The second is that even in the early stages of adolescence, you command much less attention and influence over your teen than you did at earlier stages of development. When your teen was younger, you might have, at least in the abstract, seen the value of autonomy and self-management. At the same time, until he or she reached adolescence you were playing a different role than you are now. You were actively involved in decision making day in and day out, playing a guiding role in determining the activities your child engaged in, the friends your child spent time with, the behaviors the child was expected to display, and the safety precautions the child needed to follow. You became practiced in this role and, for better or worse, made decisions in what you believed was the best interest of your child. With the onset of adolescence, however, you're increasingly yielding your role as decision maker, and your teen is gradually taking on this role. As you probably already know, this shifting of roles can be difficult. No longer are you the trusted adviser or the source of wisdom, or perhaps even the final authority. By this point, you have come to the realization that your child is growing up and that your influence is diminishing every day.

It's important not to yield to the sinking feeling that this means you have no role at all. Your teen may present the issue fairly simply: "Let me make my own decisions, trust me, and everything will be fine." You, of course, are not about to abandon your role and responsibility as a parent. So where does this leave you? With a tricky balancing act, of course. Ironically, this time when teens want more responsibility and you have less influence is also the time when your involvement is most critical. So your only choice is to find ways to work effectively *with* your teen in helping him or her make the transition to increasing decision making and autonomy.

And keep this reassuring fact in mind at all times: *While they may strongly lobby and at times fight for the opportunity to handle their lives entirely on their own, most teens realize and appreciate that parents will not simply cut them loose. While they lobby for autonomy, they do so understanding that there is a safety net that they value in place.*

They do need that safety net, more than ever, because of the degree to which adolescents are at risk. They are more heavily influenced by their peers than ever before, they have the opportunity and the means to move about their environment with fewer restrictions than they have had in the past, and developmentally they are in a risk-taking phase. This creates a pretty harrowing situation when you know that (1) adolescents sometimes make poor decisions, (2) in some cases these decisions can have serious, if not catastrophic, consequences, and (3) teens are inclined to minimize their vulnerability and dismiss your opinions about these risks.

So, this is too important a time in adolescent development for parents not to be involved. The question, then, is what will motivate your teen to work with you on negotiating his transition to independence? What motivates teens? The chance to do what adults do, make their own choices, have their opinions valued, and decide what rules will apply and how. This should come as no surprise. If choice and decision making are so important to the 4-year-old ("I do it myself!"), how much more powerful are they to the teen now that he has both the means (money, mobility, and an influential peer group) and the end of parental decision making in sight? The good news is that most of us are motivated by the same thing. We want to see our children grow up to be independent, self-sufficient adults who make sound decisions. On the face of it, then, we parents and our teenagers both want the same outcome. The devil, as they say, is in the details. While we both may want the same thing, we may not see eye to eye on how this is best accomplished, and we may not see eye to eye on what the best outcome is (for decisions about school, jobs, or friends). How often, for example, have you and your teen differed on what was "acceptable" or "okay" or "good enough"?

This may be the first time you realize that the goals you have for your child are not necessarily the goals she has for herself. If your child has weaknesses in executive skills, this may also be the first time you realize that the help you have provided in the past may no longer be as appreciated or even wanted. If, one way or the other, your teen does not "buy in," the chance of your impacting the learning and development of executive skills is seriously compromised.

Fortunately, there are a variety of ways to accomplish this buy-in. In the remainder of this chapter, we will describe the strategies and techniques you can use to increase motivation and work on executive skills, even with the reluctant or resistant teen.

Working with Your Teen to Get Buy-In

Let's suppose your teen has one or more executive skills weaknesses. Ben, for example, has a weakness in organization. If you were Ben's mother, you would have described his room as a "garbage dump" (at least to yourself, if not out loud). His return home from school is a tense moment you don't look forward to, because you've learned you have to ask him what homework he has that night or he'll discover far too late in the evening that he didn't write it down and now has to scramble to collect the assignments from classmates. He hates being "nagged" the minute he gets home. Your bank account has suffered from your having had to replace lost hockey equipment, as Ben's pride has suffered from the scorn of teammates at his constantly being late to matches because he couldn't find his stuff. Or maybe you have a daughter like Tracy, who has a problem with time management and is late not only for extracurricular activities but also for school, for assignment deadlines, and even for her own birthday party. Or do you have a son like Jason, who is weak in flexibility? You and the rest of the family could be tired of tiptoeing around Jason and doing everything you can not to surprise him because when something does not go according to his expectations or agenda, he gets angry or explodes at you.

We've found that it's important to enter into a discussion with teens about issues like these with four guidelines in mind:

1. *Be prepared to negotiate and compromise.* A willingness to engage in negotiation and compromise signals respect for a teen's autonomy and ideas and is more effective in developing executive skills than directives from a parent.

2. *Convey that your intentions are to help the teen accomplish something beneficial to him or her.* Teens are more open to help if they understand that the parents' motivation for addressing the problem is a desire to see them accomplish what is best for them—not for the parents.

3. *Focus on how the desired changes will boost your teen's independence.* Outcomes that contribute to the teen's independence and decision making will be valued more than those that emphasize parental control.

4. *Be clear in your own mind about why it's important to address the problem.* Teens will be more motivated to work on a problem that they see as important, and if you falter in your statement of the rationale, they won't be persuaded to collaborate.

Ben's mother appealed to his desire to stop her "nagging" about his homework assignments: "Ben, I know you hate being grilled the minute you walk in the door about what homework you have and where you've written down the assignment. I'd hate it too. Why don't we see if we can come up with a way for you to keep track of assignments more consistently so that when you get home we can go back to my just asking how your day went and whether anything interesting happened?"

At breakfast together one Saturday, Tracy's dad took the opportunity to try to meet his daughter halfway in solving her time management problem: "It's pretty obvious, honey, that we have really different styles when it comes to scheduling things. I know it's not fair of me to expect you to show up half an hour early for everything like I do. But when you don't plan in a way that is likely to get you places on time, you're constantly rushing and careening around, and I bet you find it hard to get anything out of what you're doing when you're always trying to catch your breath and calm down once you get there. How about we agree on something in between being 'ridiculously early,' as you call it, and being late?"

Jason's parents tried to appeal to his sadness over how some relationships that were important to him had disintegrated because of his lack of flexibility. He had lost a couple of close friends when he overreacted to their wanting to change social plans, and even his little sister, who idolized him, was beginning to avoid him because he was so touchy about her returning borrowed belongings late or not putting them back exactly where she had found them. Jason admitted that these developments hurt and agreed to try to learn to be more flexible.

Of course the parent–teen discussions were much more complicated than this, and improvements didn't drop into these families' laps just because they had all agreed to work on the teen's problems together. But when you approach the situation with these four considerations in mind, as these parents did, you will set the stage for successfully working with your teen.

Communication Don'ts

Just as there are conditions that will enhance motivation, there are types of communication that can destroy your teen's motivation or interest in working on a problem. These include the following:

1. *Stroke/kick comments.* These occur when a parent initially offers a comment such as "You did a nice job picking up your room [the stroke]," followed immediately by "I told you you could do it if you put some effort into it [the kick]."

2. *Pointing out the flaws or reasons that the problem-solving approach suggested by your teen will not work and why your solution, which you point out is based on years of experience, is better.* While this might actually be true in some cases, it does not help the teen develop her decision making unless you assume that she will happily adopt all of your problem-solving ideas. In addition, at the point that you pointed out the flaw in her approach, she stopped hearing you.

3. *Comparisons with peers or siblings.* For example, telling your teen that "Your brother, who is two years younger than you, is able to manage to keep his belongings organized, so I don't understand why you can't" does

not increase the likelihood that the problem will be solved, but it does increase the likelihood of additional sibling conflict.

4. *Approaching the problem from a position of anger or criticism.* "If I've told you once, I've told you 100 times about getting your things ready for school at night rather than in the morning! I'm sick and tired of it, and it needs to stop!"

Avoiding these don'ts does not guarantee your teen's willing participation in working on executive skills weaknesses and specific problems, but it certainly gets you closer. You might have cringed when you read through this list because you've committed some of these errors yourself. We all have, because they are simply misguided extensions of our well-intentioned efforts to teach important lessons, to offer the benefit of our experience, and, when all is said and done, to get through to a child when we feel like we've been talking to a brick wall. It takes time to make the role shift described at the beginning of this chapter.

Beginning the Process

If you're ready to begin the problem-solving process with your teen, you should be able to answer "yes" to the following questions:

1. Have you identified the problem (the executive skills weakness), the way it shows up in your teen's day-to-day functioning, and how the problem can adversely affect his future? For example, when a teen with a weakness in response inhibition listens to peers who encourage him to drive fast, he jeopardizes both his driving privileges and the safety of himself and his passengers. When a teen is late in turning in assignments, the immediate consequence is lower grades; over the long term this may affect college prospects. Meeting this first condition should put you in a better position to answer "yes" to the second question.

2. Have you conveyed to your teen, from *your* perspective, why you are worried about this problem and how it negatively impacts her life now and may impact it in the future? (This is Dick talking: My son recently said, "I remember that one of your and Mom's most persuasive arguments to me was the argument for choices. We would sit down and you would say, 'Look, Colin, we want you

to be happy. We want you to be able to make whatever choices you want. If you want to be a doctor or a lawyer, great. If you want to be a rock star or a pro baseball player, great. If you want to be a salesclerk or a construction worker, great. But we don't want you to wake up one day and decide to be something you can't because you closed off your options.'") The important part of this communication is not to browbeat your teen into believing it or saying that he believes it, or bring it up in an "I told you so" manner when he is struggling. Rather, it is simply to convey that you want what is best for him. If you have answered the first two questions affirmatively, then you've done your best to get a "yes" to the third question.

3. After you have identified the problem and explained why you are concerned about it, does your teen acknowledge it, even grudgingly, as a problem? The answer to this question doesn't just depend on how you've identified the problem or framed your concern. It also goes back to the five common adolescent response patterns we discussed in Chapter 2. Your teen's style will determine, at least in part, whether she is likely to acknowledge a problem. Whether the teen is able to acknowledge an executive skills weakness or a specific behavior that reflects that weakness determines how you will approach the motivation issue.

How to Motivate Your Teen Based on Behavioral Style

To make this discussion of executive skills and motivation more specific, let's talk about an area that is often affected by weak executive skills and is an ongoing concern for the parents of a teen: school performance.

Here's how the five styles might appear in a problem with academics:

1. "I know I have a problem that's affecting my schoolwork, but I can't manage it. Can you take care of it for me?"

2. "I have a problem that is affecting my schoolwork, and I'm open to working on it and getting help from someone [of my choosing] if that's needed."

3. "I admit that I'm having a problem and it's affecting my schoolwork. Can we work out some sort of a deal that if I work on it, I get something as a reward?"

4. "I guess I'm having a problem that's affecting my schoolwork, but I'd like to try to handle it myself."

5. "I don't think I have a problem that is affecting my schoolwork, but if so, don't worry; I'll take care of it."

From a parent's perspective, the styles of numbers 2, 3, and 4 will be the easiest to work with and motivate. Styles 1 and 5 will be more difficult.

Working with the "Take Charge" Teen. Let's start with the easier groups. The teen with style 2 comes to the situation already motivated to some degree to try to resolve the problem. Given that, your role is to talk with the teen and come to a decision about how he would like to approach or manage the problem. *The emphasis is on the teen setting the direction.* Typically, for a teen with this style, the only thing that will derail the problem solving is your trying to take a more directive role or criticizing the decision of the teen. In two-parent households, this role may be better assigned to one parent than the other if one parent has better communication with the teen. If there is the possibility of conflict with the parent, then some outside resource might be needed such as a teacher, guidance counselor, or coach. The advantage of having the other person involved is that it removes the risk of conflict with the teen and also helps the teen feel more effective and independent as a problem solver. We recommend this approach for parents who want to be in control or for parents who have ongoing conflicts with their teen.

Motivating the "Bargainer." The teen with style 3 recognizes or admits that there is a problem but doesn't feel the same urgency as the parent does to work on it or fix it. *The key to motivating this teen is to offer the teen something that she wants in exchange for something that you want.* The parent and the teen come to an agreement about some performance standard—such as the minimum grade to achieve for a particular quarter—and this is tied to earning the incentive. We have seen parents use a variety of different incentives, including cell phones or cell phone upgrades and contributions toward the purchase of desired items, including snowboards, surfboards, or even cars, depending on the expense. Some teens and some parents prefer straight cash transactions. Although we don't generally advocate cash for grades, it works for some students, and it is important for parents to keep in mind that the goal is to build habits (in this case, studying or completion of schoolwork) that ultimately will benefit the teen.

Negotiating with the "Autonomy Seeker." Teens with style 4 want to demonstrate that they are independent and can solve their own problems. Though well-intentioned, teens with this behavioral style who have executive skills weaknesses tend to have difficulty actually constructing a plan and following through on that plan. If you are a parent of a teen with this style, you want to respect the desire for independence and offer support that the teen is free to accept or not. What you cannot do, however, is simply accept your teen's statement that she will solve the problem. *This means that you and your teen must negotiate some specific performance standards (for example, on-time completion of work, a minimum grade in a particular subject), as well as a timeline for when the teen thinks they will be met.* The second part of the negotiation involves what the teen will do if she can't meet a performance standard in the time agreed on. This might mean your taking a more active planning role at that point, enlisting help from school staff, and/or tying performance to privileges. Negotiating, in advance the specifics of what will happen if the teen is not successful in her plan is very important since it helps set the agenda in both your mind and hers so that you both know what will happen next, reducing the chance of conflict or confrontation if the initial plan fails.

Supporting the "Help Seeker." Let us turn now to the more challenging behavioral styles. The teen with the first behavioral style, who feels overwhelmed by the problem and actively seeks your help, may not seem to present a major problem for you. We are used to helping our children solve problems and feel gratified when they come to us for help. What we may not appreciate at first is that jumping in to help, developing problem-solving strategies for the teen to use, or intervening with teachers does not help the teen develop the problem-solving skills needed to manage independently. You may not have to motivate this teen to take the problem seriously, but you probably *will* have to motivate her to take an active role in solving it. Your role, therefore, is to be less directive, to solicit possible problem-solving strategies from the teen, and to encourage the teen to try these strategies on her own. *Motivating this teen means providing the least amount of help necessary for her to succeed.* While initially you may be quite involved, you have to be thinking from early on about how you can be less involved and hand off some of the responsibility to the teen. For teens who lack confidence in their own ability and for their parents, this will be a slow process, and any time the teen experiences failure, she will again look to you for help.

Challenging the "Avoider." The style 5 teen's attitude is that the parent is either seeing a problem where none exists or overreacting to a problem: if only you would "relax," everything would be fine. This is the teen's attempt to deny or put the problem off. He may recognize that the problem is more serious, but may want to avoid dealing with it, or he may believe that it is not a real problem at this point and that he will be able to take care of it in time. If this is your teen, you'll need to take a more active role to compensate for your teen's laid-back attitude and avoidance of the problem. Instinctively, in attempting to take a more active role, you may become more insistent on your teen's needing to address the problem. Unfortunately, there is no reason to believe that, in and of itself, your insistence will make a significant difference to the teen. *In this case, the teen's motivation will need to come in the form of an incentive, that is, something that he wants that is of significance to him.*

In some cases, the teen with style 5 is more confrontational and insistent that her parents not meddle and therefore presents a bigger challenge for parents. As far as she is concerned, she should be able to manage her own life, make her own decisions, and decide what is and what is not a problem. These teens typically have conflicts with parents, and they tend to look at incentive systems their parents may propose as ways to manipulate their behavior. For these teens, the most powerful motivator is to be on their own and out from under parental directives and control. In this case, the motivation approach is based on something called the "Premack principle," or "Grandma's law." The idea behind Grandma's law is that if a more-preferred activity (for example, eating dessert) follows a less-preferred activity (for example, eating vegetables), then the more-preferred activity will act as a reinforcer or incentive for the less-preferred activity and increase the chance that it will happen. *For this style 5 teen, the motivational principle will always be "first–then."* Examples of this would include the following: "First finish your homework; then you can go out with your friends." "Take care of the failing grade on your math test, then you can have your driving privileges again." The assumption here is that the opportunity for the teen to be on her own (be out with friends or drive the car) is one of her most powerful motivators and is the best avenue the parent has to approach performance problems. For teens with this style of behavior, it is important (1) that the expectations and incentives be established well in advance, (2) that they be fair in the sense that the performance expectation is not unreasonable for what the incentive is, (3) that they can be earned or regained on a regular and fairly short-term basis, and (4) that parents be matter-of-fact in the way they manage the system.

Teens with this style of behavior are not necessarily going to like such a system or see it as being fair. Nonetheless, for parents who are consistent, it can be an effective system to encourage performance. For parents who use this system, there is one very important consideration in the way that it is presented to the teen—that is, it should not be presented as a negative. To say, "First [or as soon as] you finish your homework, then you can go out with your friends," is very different from saying, "If you don't finish your homework, you can't go out with your friends." The latter statement is seen as confrontational to the teen and decreases the likelihood that he will follow the direction.

The Connection between Motivation and Goals

When we want something, if we judge the goal to be realistic and believe that we have the skills or resources to achieve it, that goal serves as a motivator. With teenagers, whenever they come to us with an activity or event they would like to participate in or an object they would like to obtain, they are presenting us with a built-in motivator or incentive, and whenever possible, we should take advantage of this. In Chapter 7, we will talk specifically about the steps you can take to use your teen's specific goals as an opportunity to teach executive skills. Here we are concerned about how to use those goals as a way to motivate learning. We see teens present their parents with the following four types of goals that can be used to motivate the development of executive skills:

   1. From a parent's perspective, the ideal motivator or incentive presented as a goal by the teen is *one that is long-term and that the parent shares with the teen.* For example, the teen might want to go to college or prepare for a particular job or career. As long as the goal is realistic and within the skill set of the teen to actually achieve, this type of goal lends itself to long-term planning and provides motivation to meet the subgoals (for example, grades) along the way. You can evaluate whether the long-term motivator is working by looking to see if the teen's short-term and even day-to-day performance matches what would be needed to achieve the long-term goal.

   2. The next type of motivator or incentive is *a goal that contributes to the teen's autonomy and still has a longer-term component (for example, a few months) and will involve some planning on the part of the teen.* Included in these would be events such as getting a license, getting a car, and getting a job. All of these can involve executive skills, and getting to the end result provides a good source of

motivation. You may also see an opportunity here to use the teen's motivation to reach the goal as a way to work on another goal that you have for the teen, such as school performance. We have worked with parents who have tied school performance to getting a license, having driving privileges, and getting a job. *As long as the parental demands are realistic, some teens will be willing to strike this bargain.*

3. A third goal that may come as an incentive is more individualized. For example, a teen might want a particular cell phone or computer, a snowboard or a surfboard, or money for a trip, to name a few. Depending on the item or activity, these might be shorter- or longer-term, so if you are going to tie them to some goal you have for the teen, such as school performance, household chores, or family responsibilities, you will need a steady source of these. However, since adolescents' needs seem never-ending, you may choose to address this by making money for specific activities or events available. Tying money to specific events is important because it helps the teen engage in some planning and also helps to keep this from becoming a regular expectation on the part of teens and parents. These types of incentives are useful in a negotiation where you have a goal you would like the teen to work on that may not necessarily be the teen's goal.

4. *Not all teen goals will be acceptable to parents.* This might seem obvious, but in their quest for autonomy, teens will tend to push the envelope. (This is Dick talking: At the end of my daughter's junior year of high school, she proposed to drive herself and four friends to Montreal for a long weekend. She and her friends were only 17, and Montreal, where they knew no one, was 300 miles away. The plan was to find a place to stay when they got there, and they had about $150 each.) Our recommendation here is that you *listen and decide whether there is some part of the plan that you would consider and under what conditions you would consider it.* Teens will typically become upset if you reject their plan, but in some cases (as was the case with my daughter's proposal), parents have to say no. Doing this in as calm a manner as possible and providing reasons for rejecting the plan in terms of your concerns for the teen, while not received well at the time, leaves open the possibility for communication. You can also rest assured that your teen will be back with additional plans in the future. If there is some part of the plan that is acceptable, even with conditions, this presents another opportunity for negotiation, for your teen to experience independence with a risk that is tolerable to you, and gives you an avenue to bargain for a goal that you would like the teen to work on.

Some General Rules and Considerations for Parents about Incentives

Keeping the following principles in mind when looking for ways to help motivate your teen will increase your chances of success.

- A good incentive involves an activity or item that your teen values. With this in mind, whenever possible, start with something that your teen expresses a desire for. Doing so respects her decision making and judgment, increases her investment, and makes you seem more fair to the teen.

- If you are negotiating for some goal you have for your teen and using something that he wants as part of the bargain, make sure that the demands and incentives are matched, that is, that the "economy" is fair. If you try to get too much work for too little pay, the system will fail. If your teen insists on significant pay for minimal work, he will not meet your expectations, and you will feel taken advantage of.

- If you initially start with a long-term goal (for example, getting into college), you will have to build in shorter-term objectives and matching incentives. Teens with significant executive skills weaknesses are likely to have difficulty maintaining focus on a goal that is far in the future.

- Once you have an incentive system in place with your teen, the success of the system is determined by how often your teen actually earns the incentive. If it is less than 50% of the time, then either the incentive is not powerful enough for your teen or the demand is too great. More will be said on this below.

- The fact that you are motivated by a goal you have for your teen and believe it is best for her does not mean that your teen shares this belief. If you find yourself working harder than she is working to achieve the goal, you need to step back and ask for whom this is more important. If you realize that it is more important for you, it does not mean that you have to abandon the goal for your teen, but it does mean that you will need a more powerful incentive for her to participate, and also that you may have to make some modifications in your goal.

- Parents today provide a variety of activities and items that teens want for "free." Negotiating with them for things they want and things you want is not only desirable but important if we expect our teens to become more independent and understand that getting something of value for nothing is a rare occurrence.

Some Final Thoughts about the Connection between Effort and Motivation

Some tasks require more effort than others. This is as true for adults as it is for teens. Think about those chores at home that you put off. When we put off household chores, it is not usually because we do not have the skill to perform them. Rather, some tasks seem more effortful than others, and although we may eventually get to them, we are more likely to procrastinate about doing them or perhaps wait (or hope) that another family member will come along to take care of them. The same is true for teens; that is, some tasks will seem more effortful than others. This is not necessarily a sign that the teen does not have the skills to perform a task. If a teen has stated a desire to achieve a particular goal and has the necessary skills and an incentive to complete a task, but still hesitates or avoids it, we should consider the effortfulness of the task as an issue. The relationship of the task to the incentive is depicted in the drawing below:

Modify the relationship between the task and the incentive.

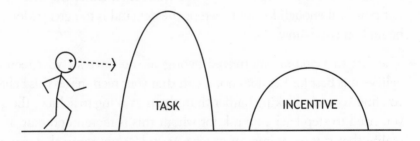

If parents expect that this is the case, then the relationship between the task and the incentive will need to be modified such that, at least in the initial stages, less is demanded. The new relationship between the task and the incentive is depicted in the next drawing:

Decrease task demands.

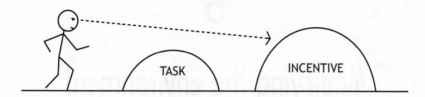

We will provide more specific detail about task modifications for this type of situation in Chapter 6, "Modifying the Environment."

6

....

Modifying the Environment

As we said earlier, there are three ways to influence the development of executive skills in your teen and to encourage the behaviors associated with those skills: The first is by motivating your teen to learn the skills or to use the skills that he has learned. We focus first on motivation because work on executive skills requires effort, and incentives of value to your teen will increase effort. When teens are unmotivated, parent–child conflict is much more likely. The second factor, and the one to which this chapter is devoted, involves modifying the environment.

By now you are familiar with the notion that from the time of your child's birth and throughout her development one of your key roles is to act as a surrogate frontal lobe. An important way that you have fulfilled this function is to help your child manage the complex and potentially dangerous situations of the adult world by lending her the benefit of your mature executive skills and your experience to create a safe environment. Within this safe environment your child, now a teenager, has been able to explore, develop, and start solving problems.

The safeguards you provided when your teen was younger fall into three broad categories: changing the way you interact with your child, changing the physical or social environment, and changing the nature of the task your child is expected to perform.

1. *Changing the way you interact with your child.* It is likely that you made and rehearsed rules or expectations before your child went into a particular situation—for example, about what types of behaviors were acceptable, what time you were leaving, or how to let the child know it was time to go. You also used verbal cues ("Remember what we talked about") and later on reminders and lists for things such as chore completion. Other ways that parents interact with their children might involve coaching or cuing them when they are in a particular situation, for example, coaching them on listening when somebody else is talking to them. You also praised your child for using good skills and debriefed him about what had happened in a particular situation, such as why a play date with a peer ended in conflict. The way you communicate or interact with your child creates an expectation, and expectations or rules are one way to modify the environment.

2. *Changing the physical or social environment.* No doubt you remember putting gates on stairs, "childproofing" a room, and even today you may use parental controls for computers and video games. You've probably also reduced distractions and stimulation by creating "quiet time" and provided organizational structures such as storage bins for toys and sports equipment and laundry baskets or hampers for dirty clothes. At one time or another, you likely changed the social environment for your child by picking and choosing playmates to avoid volatile combinations or by limiting the number of playmates at a play date.

3. *Changing the nature of tasks:* Recognizing your child's developmental limitations, you probably made chores shorter when your child was young, gave your child choices about which tasks to do or which ones to do first, and tried to make some chores more appealing by playing games like Beat the Clock for toy pickup.

In each of these ways, you took an active role in structuring your child's environment to enhance her functioning, learning, and enjoyment. While many parents make modifications like these, having a child with executive skills weaknesses you likely made more of these modifications than other parents had to. (This is Dick talking:) By the time our son reached elementary school age, my wife and I routinely structured his daily schedule on a "first–then" basis so that his less preferred and more effortful activities always preceded the fun stuff (homework came before play with friends and sax practice before TV). Once he reached adolescence and had more control over his time and access to friends, we had to expend considerably more effort to maintain these "first–then" schedules.

Environmental modifications are no less important for your teen than they were when your child was younger. In fact we would argue that in some cases they are more important, because they provide a means of risk management. We know that adolescents are more vulnerable to risk-taking activities than adults because the areas of the brain that manage motivation and impulse are not yet fully developed. Yet they have bodies that are nearly mature, and they have the social, cultural, and, in many cases, financial opportunities to engage in a variety of behaviors that they couldn't engage in as younger children.

Then there is the increased access to and influence by peers on top of their own drive for more immediate gratification. We know that teens make riskier decisions in the presence of peers, and that this occurs because the stimulation provided by peers tends to reduce a teen's use of executive skills, particularly those involving attention, emotional reactivity, impulse control, and metacognition. It's not hard to see that peer influence needs to be offset by parental support and guidance.

Unfortunately, finding appropriate opportunities and discreet ways to provide critical environmental modifications is much more difficult now that your child is older. In this chapter, we will provide you with specific strategies to implement environmental modifications in ways that are not overly intrusive or alienating to your teen. You'll find the specific strategies quite different from those you used when your child was younger, to reflect the changes in your relationship now that your child is an adolescent.

In this chapter we concentrate on changing the way you or other adults communicate and interact with your teen and changing the physical or social environment to compensate for their weak executive skills. Chapter 7, on teaching executive skills, will cover changing the nature of the task that your teen is expected to perform because the teen will participate actively in *how* the tasks will be performed (even though you will present the tasks to be done). Changing the nature of the task is therefore both an environmental modification and a skill to be learned.

Interacting with Your Teen

In terms of the ways you interact with your teen, nothing is more critical than communication. Your style of communicating is key to maintaining a positive relationship and to remaining effective as a parent. Fortunately, how you communicate is under your control.

(This is Dick talking:) We have two dogs in our family, one of which our daughter identifies as hers, because she contributed a substantial part of her savings to buy it and chose the dog. However, if ownership is based on time and interaction with the dog (walking, feeding, cleaning up), the dog belongs to my wife and me. We do have an informal agreement with my daughter about exercising the dog, which she is supposed to do on an every-other-day basis. My wife and I like to walk the dog, so we are insistent about the agreement only if we are both busy over consecutive days. If our daughter forgets, a reminder may or may not be effective. After a day or two of her forgetting, my annoyance builds, and my irritation is readily identifiable by my vocal intonation and the words I choose. While the result is usually that my daughter will take the dog out, we have had some arguments, and it is not always a happy event for the dog. At the same time, I am aware that a less confrontational approach usually leads to the same outcome and leaves me, my daughter, and the dog in a happier frame of mind. So for me the best approach is to say, "Shan, we haven't been able to take the dog out for _____ days. She needs some company, and I need you to take her out before [whatever event is on her schedule]." When I approach it in this way, she is as likely to follow through as she is with the other type of communication, and when she does not, my fallback is to remind her that before she goes out to _____, she needs to take the dog out. While she may express some irritation at this, it is certainly less, and the dog and I are happier. In approaching the problem this way, we try to follow the four guidelines for discussing issues with teens presented in Chapter 5. If this were a task or chore that my wife and I had more investment in my daughter completing (for example, being on time with schoolwork, managing or spending money), we would be more systematic in our approach.

The point here is simple. We control the way we approach the situation and by doing so elicit a different behavior from our daughter. For all of us as parents, the expectations, directions, and rules involved in important situations provide structure for the behavior of our teens, and the outcomes are significantly influenced by the style we use to communicate that information.

Communication Strategies

In their book *Defiant Teens*, Russell Barkley, Gwenyth Edwards, and Arthur Robin suggest four areas that can significantly impact adult–teen interactions. The first area involves *dos and don'ts for communication* that enhance parent–teen cooperation. The following lists are adapted from their work.

Don'ts	Dos
Use insults.	State the issue.
Interrupt.	Take turns.
Criticize.	Note good and bad.
Get defensive.	Calmly disagree.
Give lectures.	Say it short and straight.
Get distracted.	Pay attention.
Use sarcasm.	Talk in a normal tone.
Go silent.	Say what you feel.
Yell.	Accept responsibility.
Swear.	Use emphatic but respectful language.

To these, we would add some general principles of effective communication:

1. Teens are not always ready or in the mood to talk, and when a parent tries to force the issue, communication is less likely. On the other hand, when your teen is ready to talk, try to make yourself available to listen, even when it may not be convenient. If you're not available, offer a specific time when you can talk. (This is Dick talking:) My daughter and I communicate frequently by text or phone. We agreed on an arrangement that when I cannot interrupt a meeting I am in to speak with her, I will text the letter *L*, which means that I can't talk right now but will call as soon as I can, and she uses the same letter if she cannot be interrupted by my text or phone call.

2. Use active listening. Active listening involves paying attention to what your teen is saying, using gestures to indicate that you understand, and from time to time demonstrating that you understand by briefly paraphrasing the gist of what the teen is saying. Listening is key. Try to avoid the urge to immediately offer an opinion, a judgment, or a solution to what you see as a problem. When the situation calls for it, honestly express how you feel, whether it is positive or negative, without being hurtful or insulting. (This is Dick again:) Amy, the daughter of a friend of ours, was frustrated when her mother didn't always listen in a way the girl thought was helpful, so she presented her mother with the following list of "my discussion types."

- "Storyteller"—I tell my story and you listen but don't solve the problem.
- "Suggestory"—I explain my story, then you listen and give suggestions *at the end*.
- "Detective"—I explain my problem, give a few possible solutions, and ask for a few solutions from you.
- "Along the way"—I explain my story and along the way you give advice and/or suggestions.
- "Conversation"—We have a regular, back-and-forth discussion.

While these may not be the same for all discussions, we offer them to parents as a way to understand that when your teen comes to talk with you, she will have different needs at different times. Initially, we recommend that parents always start with the "storyteller" approach—that is, the teen talks and you listen.

3. Negotiate whenever you can and save the nonnegotiables for situations that are important. At a time when there is no pending issue or conflict and you both are calm and have time to talk, let your teen know that issues will come up and you will do your best to hear and respect his point of view and negotiate or compromise whenever possible. There are also times when, as a parent, you will not be able to compromise or negotiate.

4. Avoid the *knee-jerk "no"* to any request that your teen makes. "No" needs to remain in your vocabulary, but use it judiciously and be prepared to present your reasons.

We will have more to say about these communication strategies below, when we discuss how parents can give effective directions to teens.

Unreasonable Beliefs

A second factor impacting parent–teen communication, according to Barkley and his colleagues, involves *unreasonable parental beliefs and expectations*. To help you better understand and live with your teen's behavior and improve communication, we offer our adaptation of the four unreasonable beliefs and expectations discussed in *Defiant Teens*.

1. *Teens should make few mistakes and always follow parental rules and expectations.* Some parents get quite upset over a missed homework assignment, a low grade on a test, an incomplete chore, or a "bad attitude." Unless the problem is recurring and clearly has a negative impact on home or school performance, assume that these things will happen from time to time and are a typical part of a teenager's development.

2. *When we give teenagers too much freedom, they will make catastrophic errors and ruin their lives.* While there is no "one size fits all" guideline for how much freedom to give a teen, we offer guidelines below to manage catastrophic risks. At the same time, the freedom to make decisions *and* mistakes is how teens learn and become responsible adults. If we want our teens to become good decision makers and problem solvers, we must take the risk of letting *them* take the risk.

3. *Teens misbehave in a deliberate attempt to annoy us or as payback for some consequence we have imposed.* While this may happen from time to time, most of the limit testing that teens engage in involves a desire for independence and a chance to guide their own lives and is not intended as a way to punish parents.

4. *Teens should express appreciation for all that their parents have done for them.* Teens, particularly the younger ones, are focused on themselves and the things that are important in their world, namely their peers. As is the case with a number of aspects of teen development (like increased self-discipline and good judgment), parents may have to wait until late adolescence, young adulthood, or longer for expressions of appreciation.

In communicating with your teen, periodically ask yourself about your own beliefs and expectations: Are you being realistic in the way you're approaching your teen about particular behaviors or situations?

Giving Effective Directions

The third key element for parents in parent–teen communication is *how to give effective directives or communicate expectations*. If you expect your teen to listen to you, the following guidelines, adopted and modified from Barkley and his colleagues, are key.

1. *Make sure you mean it!* This means you do not give a direction that you do not intend to see either completed or followed up with a consequence if it is not completed. Again, this may seem self-evident, but much of what parents say to their teens in the form of directions is simply heard as "noise" by the teen because either there is no follow-up or the follow-up comes hours or days later. Whenever possible, make the directions specific and make eye contact with your teen when the direction is given. For example, if your teen is in his room and you are downstairs and holler upstairs, "Jack, you need to clean your room [pick up your dishes, mow the lawn, walk the dog, etc.]" and say nothing beyond that, the likelihood that the direction will be followed is pretty low. If instead you walk upstairs or call Jack downstairs, make eye contact, and say, "I need you to put the dirty clothes on the floor in your room in the laundry basket and bring it down before you go out with your friends," you have increased the likelihood that Jack heard what you had to say and has a time frame for your expectation for his getting it done. It also allows you to set the possible consequence by asking Jack, when he is ready to go out with his friends, if he has completed the task. If he has not, you are in the position to say, "As soon as you do that, you can go out." When you don't follow up, you encourage your teen not to listen.

2. *Do not present a direction or expectation as a question or favor.* Give the direction directly and in a businesslike tone. In this situation, parents often anticipate some resistance to the direction and as a result present the direction with an edge of irritability or anger, perhaps because the direction has been ignored before. As we said earlier, this does not increase the effectiveness of the direction and in fact makes it more likely that the parent and teen will end up in some sort of verbal conflict. Parents also will phrase directions as questions ("Would/could you clean your room?") when in fact they are not presenting the question as a choice. If you do want to give your teen a legitimate choice ("Would you like to pick up your room before or after dinner?"), the question format is fine. If your intent is not to present a choice, give the direction as a statement.

3. *Do not give too many directions at once.* Since parent–teen contact is often fleeting, parents may feel the need to present a list of directions or expectations. This is typically a source of considerable irritability to teens, who see it as "piling on." Try to limit the directions to one or two at a time.

4. *Tell your teen what to do rather than what not to do.* Telling your teen what specifically you want her to do sets up an expectation in her mind for the next step to follow. Telling a teen what not to do does not provide him with a concrete behavior to work toward.

5. *Avoid competing distractions when giving your teen directions.* Because contact with teens is fleeting and they are frequently engaged in some activity (texting, Facebook, phone, TV), parents make the mistake of trying to give a direction while teens are engaged in another activity. When something more entertaining is going on (and almost anything is more entertaining than your parent telling you what to do!), parent directions are not heard. This is the case even if the teen acknowledges having heard the parent. Who among us hasn't mastered the art of telling a person we have heard him when in fact we are focused on something else? If your direction is going to be effective, you need to have your teen's undivided, even if brief, attention. If you are not sure the teen heard you, have her paraphrase, but use this sparingly.

A related issue involves the timing of parent directions. When your teen is just arriving home, on his way out the door, about to go to sleep, or just waking up, the first words out of your mouth should not be about something you want done. If your son is on his way out the door or on his way to bed, there is no purpose in stating the expectation unless you are prepared to interfere with the completion of either of those activities until the expectation is met, since it will have to be restated at a time when your son is more likely to be able to meet the expectation. The only exceptions to this rule are quick reminders about behavioral expectations with friends, curfews, brushing teeth before bed, and other things that are part of the activity the teen is going to engage in. When your teen is coming in from an activity or event, greeting him first and giving him a chance to talk about what he was doing avoids the "transition shock" of being hit with a nonpreferred activity as soon as he comes in the door. Similarly, wake-up time for teens in the morning is a slow and perhaps irritable process, so parent directions at that point often only make this a stressful time of day.

Rules and Expectations

You can make a few general and reliable assumptions about rules and expectations for adolescents. By this point you realize that the drive for independence, the opportunity for your teenager to make her own decisions and choices, is a powerful one. In the absence of rules and expectations, of agendas set by parents, teens will naturally fill the void with their own expectations and agendas. Privacy plays a significant role in teens' independence. Since their agendas are likely to be set according to the values and expectations of their peers, you may not know what their plans or expectations are until you present your own, only to discover that they have already filled the void. For many teens, once they have established an expectation they hold tight to it, and if a parent has a different expectation the result will be a conflict. While there is no way to prevent this from happening all the time, our advice is to put your rules and expectations on the table early and review them regularly.

Guidelines for Setting Rules

Beyond this, a few other guidelines can help you set rules effectively:

1. Limit the number of rules you have and keep in mind that the rules you set are intended to act as a limit for your teen in your absence and protect him from risks that he might otherwise take.

2. Try to develop rules that cover a range of situations but are at the same time specific and not open to interpretation. For example, "Be home at a reasonable hour" is not an effective rule, but "Be home at 12 o'clock" is.

3. Decide in advance on any exceptions to the rule. For example, if midnight is the curfew, is that an absolute deadline, or will you accept some flexibility, for example, plus or minus 15 minutes? While you don't want to be inflexible, exceptions undermine rules and should be accepted only sparingly.

4. If you expect rules to be followed, make sure consequences are associated with not following them and that these are stated in advance.

5. Whenever possible, rely on the rules and consequences that other authorities (Internet service providers, schools, teachers, towns, states, etc.) have instituted and review these with your teen.

Areas That Call for Rules

Based on interviews with parents and teenagers, we recommend that you consider rules for the following areas:

1. *Curfew.* This is an area that teens will want to negotiate and that will change as they age. There will be some variation to take into consideration: school versus weekend nights and special events. Be sure to have a nonnegotiable bottom line.

2. *Location.* Know approximately where your teen is and when he is making a major location change, such as going from a friend's house to the mall or a different friend's house.

3. *Whom your teen is with.* This is not meant to be a minute-by-minute accurate accounting of everyone the teen interacts with, but a general idea of whom she will be spending her time with. As part of this, we would recommend having the cell phone numbers of close friends in case, for some reason, you can't reach your own teen. This is primarily for emergencies and not for use when your teen does not respond to your first phone call or text message.

4. *Contact with friends' parents.* When your teen is planning a sleepover, attending a house party, taking a trip to a beach or lake house, or the like, it is important that you speak with the parents of the teen hosting the event to ensure that they know it is happening and that they will in fact be there. When an overnight stay is involved, the expectation is that your teen remains at the house unless he notifies that parent that he is leaving, and the parent in turn agrees to notify you.

5. *Acceptable use of electronic/social media.* This includes information that your teen is posting about herself or peers, websites she frequents, and information she downloads.

6. *Avoidance of alcohol, drugs, and, depending on your personal beliefs, sex (or in any case, unprotected sex).* With regard to alcohol and drugs, schools and/or school athletic departments may reinforce these rules by requiring students to sign contracts prohibiting use or being in the presence of it. (This is Dick talking: We have found it necessary to extend the alcohol and drugs rule to situations where parents of another teen have felt that provision of alcohol to underage teens was acceptable, since they were present to monitor.) Make sure your teen understands that *your* rules, not those of friends *or* their parents, govern these topics.

7. *People, places, and situations that are off limits.*

8. *Avoidance of other activities that are illegal or would be considered unethical.*

From a teen's perspective most of what goes on in his life, unless he chooses to tell you, is none of your business. Your role as a parent is to decide in advance and to communicate to the teen what is your business. Fair areas of inquiry include:

- Information about performance in school

- Information about driving habits

- Information about where the teen is spending time and with whom

- Any involvement or suspected involvement with alcohol or drugs

- If the teen is involved in sexual activity, information about unprotected sex, given the risks of sexually transmitted diseases and pregnancy and the potential emotional toll of premature sexual relationships

Stating this to teens does not guarantee that they will readily offer information, but it does let them know that in your role as a parent you will seek out information regarding these areas.

Making Consequences Effective

Consequences, like rules, are a significant environmental modification that you control, and they can have an important impact on your teen's behavior. In their program for defiant teens, Barkley and his colleagues indicate that consequences should have six characteristics: specificity, immediacy, consistency, meaningfulness, frequency, and balance.

Specificity. As with rules, consequences need to be specific. Avoid vague threats such as "You'll regret it if you're not home on time." State a consequence such as "If you're late by 30 minutes or less, you'll need to come home an hour earlier tomorrow night. If you're more than a half-hour late, you will lose your privilege of going out tomorrow night." Related to specificity, parents should use consequences that are logically related to the rule that is broken. For example, unsafe driving leads to the loss of driving privileges. Loss or destruction of property leads to replacement or financial restitution. Inaccurate information about location or activities leads to loss of participation.

Immediacy. Consequences have their most powerful effect when they occur immediately. For example, if a chore or a task such as homework needs to be completed prior to a teen's engaging in a preferred activity, access to that activity should occur only when the required activity has been completed. This is likely to require direct checking by you rather than simply taking your teen's word for it. If direct checking is not possible (for example, you are not home), then when you discover the task was not completed, the teen's preferred activity should be interrupted at that point until the task is complete. In other cases, such as breaking curfew, immediate consequences are not possible, but the consequence should occur at the next opportunity that the teen has for that privilege.

Consistency. This principle applies both to the rules that are made and to how they are applied. Rules should not vary according to who is doing the parenting (mother, father, grandparents, etc.), what type of mood they are in, or what the situation is (for example, if peers, family friends, or extended family are present). If teens see that consequences vary according to who is parenting or what the situation is, the effectiveness of the consequence and the rule is undermined. In a similar way, inconsistent application of a consequence over time undermines the rule. For example, if a teen's coming in after an agreed-upon time sometimes results in a consequence and other times is ignored, the rule is more likely to be broken.

Meaningfulness. Whether for negative or positive behavior, consequences should be meaningful, that is, related to the subject of the rule. Take curfew as an example. If a teen violates curfew, it makes sense to impose a consequence of setting an earlier curfew until the teen adheres to the rule. A teen who consistently obeys a curfew and is rewarded with a later curfew will see this as a meaningful, positive consequence. For teens, any positive consequence that is tied to the opportunity for increased independence, decision making, and control over choices will be valued.

Frequency. In terms of negative consequences, frequency is related to consistency. If you've given a rule or a direction that the teen does not follow, a consequence should always follow. If you rely on restating or threatening a consequence but you don't regularly deliver it, your teen is unlikely to follow rules and directions.

Balance. Balance has two meanings. The first relates to fairness, ensuring that negative consequences are in proportion to the offense. If a teen occasionally misses curfew, establishing an earlier curfew for the next night out is a balanced response. Restricting the teen to the home for a week is not. Major consequences like extended restriction to the home should be saved for major offenses. Balance also relates to positive and negative consequences. *We know from the behavioral change literature that when positive comments outweigh negative comments by a ratio of three to one or more, an increase in positive behavior is likely.* When negative consequences outweigh positive consequences, teens lose motivation to follow the rules or meet expectations. When teens have "nothing left to lose," parents have little, if any, ability left to influence behavior.

The Use of Outside Experts

Throughout your child's life, from infancy through preadolescence or perhaps early adolescence, you, as parent, fulfill the primary role as advice giver and resident expert. You show your child how to use utensils, get dressed, brush her teeth, prepare food, fix machinery or broken objects, solve problems with friends, and so forth. You show your child how to throw, kick, or catch a ball. You help her with their homework, and you talk with her teachers, and when the child needs help, she comes to you with the expectation that you will be able to answer her question, find an answer for her, or help solve her problem. You do all of these things in the service of your child's becoming more self-reliant and independent.

The first indication that you may be displaced or replaced as your teenager's resident expert probably comes from teachers or coaches. When your child says to you, "That's not how my coach showed me to do it" or "That's not what my teacher said we were supposed to do," it is a reminder that in certain areas you are no longer the expert. Given the ever-increasing technological sophistication of children and the wealth of information available, it's likely that future parents will play a diminished role as advice givers and experts. This is especially true for adolescents who are looking to establish themselves as independent decision makers and who more and more want to rely on themselves and their friends for information and advice. At the same time, parents continue to handle much of what are considered to be adult affairs, including financial and tax management, health and automobile insurance, legal affairs, and medical treatment. For a young child, these things are "behind the scenes," and the child is either unaware of or unable to understand them.

If we want our teens to be independent and competent young adults, we should introduce them to these affairs. For example, involving your teen in household budgets and informing the teen about expenditures, including groceries, utilities, car payments, rent, and mortgages, gives him a sense that he is assuming a more adult role in the family. Taking this one step further and letting him be directly involved with experts gives him a different perspective on how the real world operates and begins to build a skill set that the teen will require over time. If he wants to have some control over his own finances, have him talk with managers in local banks as a prelude to setting up his own accounts. If cars need to be inspected or repaired, let your teen take the car in and interact directly with service managers. If he has questions about legal matters, schedule a brief meeting with an attorney who can answer his questions. If there are health concerns or if there is health information you would like your teen to be aware of, set up appointments with doctors, dentists, or nurse practitioners so that the teen can meet with them. In short, if there is any situation with which your teen as a young adult will need to be familiar, introduce him to the people who are experts in those areas and let your teen interact independently with them.

For teens with executive skills weaknesses, if you're introducing this independent use of experts for the first time, you probably need to follow up with the expert (auto mechanic, doctor, dentist, bank manager) to ensure that any information conveyed to the teen that involves you actually gets to you. You don't want to find out 3 months later that the car needs brakes or that there's a prescription for antibiotics sitting (unfilled) on your son's bedroom floor. Also, in using certain kinds of experts, make sure you can live with the information they give to the teen. Doctors may have frank discussions about sexual behaviors, and lawyers may offer advice about what search rights police do and do not have.

Physical Modifications

The last category of environmental modifications you can provide that will help guide the behavior of your adolescent until she has developed her own executive skills involves physical and technological modifications to the environment. One of the major categories involves communication and monitoring. When our children are very young, we want to be able to see and hear them. To accomplish this we provide playpens, gates, or fenced-in areas, or we use baby monitors. When they are a little bit older, we let them travel distances by taking them there or check to make sure that they got there and that some other adult is in charge. Thus we reassure ourselves of our children's safety by having some line of communication to them.

In adolescence, when they have significantly increased freedom to move about the environment, cell phones play that role and usually represent the best option that parents have of maintaining an open line of communication with their teens. Cell phones can be used simply as communication devices where parents or teens can initiate the communication, or they can be used to provide ongoing and accurate information about location using built-in GPS systems. How parents choose to use these devices depends on the extent to which they want to rely on their teen's ability to manage her behavior independently. We have provided information about a range of cell phone applications that can be used for communication and monitoring purposes in the Resources at the end of the book.

A second type of communication and monitoring device involves cars. There is a range of devices that will provide information not only about vehicle location but also about driving habits, including speed, braking maneuvers, and so forth. These are listed separately in the Resources section.

A third type of technological application involves more active management of teen behavior. In terms of phone applications, it is now possible to establish area perimeters and have parents notified if teens go beyond these particular areas. Some automobile models come equipped with systems that automatically disable cell phone use while the car is moving, and there are also software applications that can be added to automobiles to accomplish similar functions. There are also active driving systems that will limit the speed of cars or provide in-car feedback when teens engage in dangerous driving habits.

Given the technological savvy of most adolescents, use of environmental modifications like parental controls is more complicated. But these, as well as technology parents can use to monitor Internet use, continue to be available. In terms of decreasing catastrophic risk, one of the most important environmental modifications involves decisions about the types of vehicles that teenagers drive. The accident and injury statistics involving young teenage drivers range from sobering to frightening, depending on whether you have a teen currently driving or not. According to the Centers for Disease Control (statistics for 2009), car crashes are the leading cause of death among 16- to 19-year-olds annually, with approximately 3,000 deaths and 350,000 injuries. Teens are four times more likely to crash than older drivers. Given these facts, teenagers should drive the safest car that you can afford. Whenever possible, at a minimum teenagers should be driving cars that are equipped with antilock brakes and front, side, and side-curtain airbags. Since teen drivers nationwide are involved in the highest percentage of automobile accidents, putting your teen in a safe vehicle is simply one of the wisest decisions you can make.

Since we are on the issue of safety, one other major environmental modification that has a significant impact on injury prevention for teens is using helmets. If your teen skis, snowboards, skateboards, or rides a bike, helmet use will significantly decrease the likelihood of brain injury.

The remainder of the physical modifications we would recommend relate to other areas of executive skill weakness. The modifications include the following:

- Alarm clocks

- Organizing systems for study materials and room keeping

- Wall and/or desk calendars

- Whiteboards for scheduled or special events

There may well be a number of others, but you get the idea. We should also note that with any of the environmental modifications just described it is important that you involve your teen in the decision making about the modification and, if you have a specific reason for using something that is invasive from the teen's perspective (for example, GPS monitoring systems), that you provide a clear rationale for its use. Having said this, you can still expect that your teen will find your suggested environmental modification intrusive. Remember, teens are coming from the perspective that they can manage on their own. How intrusive a modification feels—and how defensive they get—depends on a number of factors, including what their personal style is: The "take charge teen" will manage the suggestion less defensively than the "avoider." Beyond that, your presentation of the problem and proposed solution are likely to be received more calmly if you've used the principles from Chapter 4 and the rules for discussion in Chapter 5. The following vignette deals with a frequent and very annoying problem for parents.

Hannah didn't know what to do with her son Alex. He was a good kid; he had a great sense of humor, was a good student, and got along with his family surprisingly well for a teenager. Hannah's problem was Alex's sense of responsibility, or lack thereof, when it came to picking up after himself. It was the kind of behavior that might have been funny if it were part of a teen coming-of-age comedy, but this movie never ended. Dirty clothes were everywhere; jackets and shoes littered the living room floor. The bathroom floor was apparently an altar on which offerings to the god of sweaty gym clothes and dirty socks sat for days. Even when Alex did do laundry, he would forget about it and then take clean items, one at a time, out of the dryer as though it were an auxiliary dresser. But the worst of his transgressions by far involved dirty dishes. Cereal bowls left on the counter along with a half carton of milk were a given. But Alex seemed to have the ability to eat in every part of the house and then leave the dish wherever it was most convenient. Plates went under the bed; coffee cups and spoons were inevitably left on surfaces most receptive to permanent Rorschach stains. It seemed like Hannah went as often to Alex's computer desk to look for silverware as she did to the drawer where it belonged.

Hannah hadn't simply put up with it either. Alex had been harassed, harangued, and otherwise hassled by Hannah and her boyfriend Marcus as far back as they could remember. But they couldn't think of an effective way to control how Alex used communal items. Hannah was at her wit's end. She couldn't believe something like this was driving her crazy, but it was, and it was adding totally unnecessary tension to their relationship.

One evening, after Hannah had gone to Alex's room to scold him and returned balancing dishes like a cartoon character, she and Marcus sat down to brainstorm.

"What if . . . we made him eat everything off a Frisbee with a toy beach shovel, you know, teach him a lesson?" Marcus said. Hannah punched him on the shoulder. "Har har har. I'm not even sure that would deter him. But seriously, I have no idea how to tackle this."

"Well, I think first we need to make it clear that we can't live like this. Then I think we need to come up with some sort of system that teaches him how to pick up."

After some discussion, they came up with a few ideas. The next day when Alex came home from school, Hannah had him sit down with her and Marcus to tell him what the plan was.

"Alex, honey, we really can't live like this anymore. The house is constantly a mess, and most of it seems to be your stuff. I understand that a dish here or some shorts there doesn't seem like a lot, but it adds up, and what's worse for me is that I can't see the light at the end of the tunnel. So, starting now, here's what we're going to do."

Hannah grabbed a bag on the floor beside her and set it on the table. Out of it she pulled out two each of ceramic bowls, plates, and silverware, all in matching blue tones.

"These are your dishes. No one else will use them, and you won't use anything else. If I find that you've been using our dishes and leaving them out, you get a warning. Three warnings and you spend a weekend night in

*the house doing chores. Also, we will ask that you not eat in your room. I
know that might sound strange, but if you want a snack and some privacy,
use the living room; you know Marcus and I don't spend much time there."*

Alex laughed. "This is a joke, right? I mean how crazy does this sound
to you?"

Hannah responded, "Very. It sounds insane. But I feel like we have
no other option. We've been picking up after you for years, thinking that as
you got older you would learn to do it for yourself. And I don't mean leaving something out once in a while. I mean that it is a consistent and serious
problem. We're always running out of silverware, picking up after you, even
finding food that was starting to rot. I can't tolerate that."

Alex thought about that for a minute, then nodded slowly. "Okay, I
can get that. But you guys know this can't go on forever either, right?"

"We know, and we don't want to make you feel unwelcome in your
own home. As we see that you are able to maintain your own set of dishes,
we will allow you back into our supply, but the no-food-in-your-room rule
is permanent; we feel it's an issue of cleanliness."

Alex sighed. "Okay, fine."

"On the issue of laundry: Sometimes you get a load through and then
leave it in the dryer, nibbling off the load when you need something. From
now on, here's what we're going to do; if a load of your laundry has been
sitting in the dryer too long, I will take it hostage, and you won't get it back
until you do another load. If this doesn't work, than we will take something
else, like your Xbox controllers."

"NOOO!" Alex jokingly (but also seriously) wailed.

"I know, terrifying."

"Okay, I can work with this. But as far as food in my room is concerned, we need to come to an agreement. It's easy to say that I can just 'go
somewhere else' for privacy, but there's only one room in this house that's
really mine. How about this? Prepackaged snacks and drinks in my room,
and I empty the trashcan every other day. No dishes."

Hannah looked at her son and smiled just for a second. "Okay, we got
a deal. No junk food, though."

"No junk food."

7

Teaching Executive Skills

Incentives and other motivational strategies outlined in the previous chapter can help teens develop more effective executive skills as long as they know how to use the skill in question and simply need to be prodded to use it or practice it. For a student who's chronically late for school, for instance, knowing that he can drive to school only if he leaves the house by a certain time may by itself persuade him to improve his time management skills by getting up promptly when the alarm goes off and going through his morning routine efficiently. Or for a teen with problems with emotional control, letting her know that the trip to the mall with friends on Saturday is contingent on her not blowing her stack with her younger sister between Friday evening and Saturday afternoon may help her practice self-restraint when she finds out Friday night that her sister has borrowed a favorite piece of clothing without permission. In both these cases, the incentive (access to the family car or a trip to the mall) is sufficient to prod the teenager to implement a plan or a procedure that will improve the executive skill in question.

For many teens with executive skills weaknesses, however, being *motivated* is not enough, because they *genuinely do not know how to do* what we (and they) want them to do. The youngster with time management problems, for instance, may have no idea how to structure his time to ensure he can get out the door on time (for example, by getting his backpack ready the night before, selecting the clothes he's going to wear, or knowing how to pull himself back to task when something on television catches his eye). Or the girl with problems with emotional control may not have learned that there are other options besides screaming at her sister (for example, calming down and counting to 20 before speaking, writing her a note rather than yelling at her, or enlisting a parent to help with solving a seemingly intractable problem).

For parents who want to help their teenagers develop executive skills, there is no "one size fits all" approach or formula. In this chapter, we describe three different situations that you may encounter and how these present opportunities to work on executive skills with your teen. The first involves directly teaching the skill when the two of you are in agreement that the skill needs to be built and the teen is willing to work with you. The other, more complicated situations are those where *you* see the glaring skill deficit, but your child either doesn't acknowledge it or doesn't think it's worth trying to correct ("Who cares if I'm late? My friends have adjusted and just expect that I will always show up about 30 minutes after I said I would," or "I wouldn't have a problem controlling my temper if my sister didn't keep taking my things without asking!"). We'll show you how to teach a skill by working on a goal (or incentive) that your teen wants. We'll also show you how to enlist your teen's participation in activities of daily living required by all families—such as shopping, appointments, and money management—as a way to learn executive skills. Both you and your teen will feel more confident in the teen's ability to manage independently when she can handle these routine tasks successfully.

In all these cases, one guiding principle rises above all others: *involve your teen at every step of the way.* Your child is too old to be told what to do (at least without causing repercussions that could undermine the process) and old enough to bring both good ideas to the table, as well as the self-knowledge to identify the strategies that have a shot at working and those that probably need to be rejected out of hand. We will remind you of this as we move through this chapter, but it's important enough to stress at the outset.

Directly Teaching Executive Skills

As stated earlier, about 5% of teenagers with executive skills weaknesses seem to know they have a deficit and are willing to work with a parent to address the problem. Another 20 percent know they have a deficit and can be persuaded through the use of a reinforcer or incentive to work with a parent (or some other adult) to address the problem. So the steps described below will help 25% of teenagers work with an adult to create a plan that has a high chance of success. Here are the steps to follow to create the plan:

Step 1: Identify the Problem Behavior You Want to Work On

There are two parts to this step. First, together with your teen, identify the specific executive skills weakness and then identify the problem situation in which the weakness manifests itself. Let's use the examples from the beginning of the chapter:

Executive skills weakness: Time management.

Problem situation: Jake is routinely late for school in the morning (or gets out the door on time only with frequent nagging and reminders from his parents).

Executive skills weakness: Emotional control.

Problem situation: Maxine frequently loses her temper with her sister, resulting in loud shouting matches.

Why is it important to identify the executive skill and not just the problem situation? For two reasons. First of all, it reminds us that we are truly talking about a missing or deficient skill rather than just a problem situation that could be avoided if the teen would only *try harder.* Second, it helps us think about how the skill deficit might show up in other problem situations so that we can keep those in mind while devising the teaching strategy and perhaps help the teen apply the strategy to those situations as well (known in the behavioral literature as *building in generalization*).

How do you decide which executive skills and problem situations to start with? Here are some types of information that might help you answer this question:

• *Your child's assessment of areas of weakness that are worth tackling.* Ask what your teen sees as the most pressing problem. Since this might be a difficult discussion, we suggest you begin by highlighting your child's strengths (identified in the Chapter 2 questionnaire)—be sincere and provide enough details about how you see the strength having a positive impact so that your teen knows you're being genuine. Ask if the teen wants to add anything to the strengths discussion before moving on to address problems. Then look at the weak executive skills and ask if your teen can identify problem situations that are an impediment to success in school or other important life activities.

• *The highest scores on the Executive Skills Questionnaire* in Chapter 2. These point to the weakest skills, which might be a place to start.

• *Your own informal observations* of the daily or weekly predicaments your child finds herself in that seem to be associated with a weak executive skill. If your daughter is routinely losing points for late homework assignments because she forgot them or couldn't manage her time well enough to complete them by the deadline, then that may be a reasonable focus for an intervention. If your son is getting in trouble with teachers for talking back to them to the point where he is earning detentions, that may be the place to start.

• *Feedback from teachers* about chronic problems your child displays. Careless mistakes on tests or papers, being unwilling to take risks for fear of making mistakes, getting poor grades on tests due to not studying enough or studying the wrong material, handing in projects with pieces missing, producing poor-quality work when your teen seems capable of more . . . these are the problems teachers often bring up on report cards or in parent conferences. If you've been hearing about them for a while or they occur with more than one teacher or subject, they may be reasonable targets for intervention.

• *Your own assessment of what the most pressing problem is.* If your teen identified numerous weak skills on the Chapter 2 questionnaire, all of which are associated with many different problem situations, how do you select one to target? First, which problem situation is getting your child in the hottest water right now? If he's failing classes, burning bridges with friends, teachers, coaches, or employers, or putting himself at risk by making impulsive decisions, you may want to focus on the skill deficits underlying these problems. With these "hot water" situations, catastrophic risks should take priority. An alternative approach is to take the long view: of all the skill deficits or problem situations your child is coping with, which one is likely to have the biggest impact down the road? It may be helpful to finish the following sentence: *By the time my child graduates from high school I hope he/she will be able to* _____. (This is Peg talking:) When I did this exercise when my own son was beginning high school, it helped me decide that I wanted to work on helping him get his homework done and handed in on time because I felt this translated into critical future workplace skills of fulfilling task obligations and meeting deadlines. I decided to tolerate his messy bedroom because it was harder to see how this might impact an important area of life functioning down the road.

If you're lucky, the information from all these sources will converge. Now see if you and your teen can distill everything into two critical pieces of information: the executive skills weakness and the target problem situation. Use the space below to write down one or two executive skills weaknesses your teen is willing to work on and the problem situations in which those weaknesses arise.

Executive skills weakness: _____

Problem situation: _____

_____

_____

Executive skills weakness: _____

Problem situation: _____

_____

_____

Step 2: Set a Goal

The goal is most often a positive restatement of the problem behavior. Here are possible goals for the two examples listed above.

> *Goal:* Jake will get to school on time without parental reminders. (Note: Obviously we're not talking literally about *no* reminders, but whereas reminders are now the rule, when the goal is met, they will be the exception.)
>
> *Goal:* Maxine will handle conflicts with her sister without raising her voice or using unkind language.

Well-defined goals usually describe behavior that can be seen or heard or otherwise verified. The two goals above satisfy this condition. Now you try it for the problem situations you've identified:

Goal: _____

_____

Goal: _____

_____

Step 3: Establish a Way to Show Progress

If you've identified a problem situation that is chronic and more than mildly irritating, achieving your goal will take time, so it's wise to set interim goals or figure out how to show that progress is being made. Since this whole process is a collaborative effort, ask your teen for ideas about how you'll know when progress is being made. If she draws a blank, one of the ideas below might be worth trying. However you monitor progress, it's essential that both of you be sure from the outset about exactly what constitutes progress or success.

Here are two measurement possibilities:

1. *Find some way to count behaviors.* Behaviors that can be counted include:

   - numbers of reminders needed before the task is begun or done
   - amount of time between when the teen *says* he will do something and the time he actually starts doing it
   - number of times the youngster engages in the problem behavior (if you're counting negative behaviors) or the goal behavior (if you're counting positive behaviors, which is typically the preferred approach)
   - length of time something lasts (e.g., the amount of time spent studying for a test, working on a homework assignment, or completing a chore).

   In the examples above, behaviors that might be counted include the number of days the student arrives late to school, the number of reminders needed to get him out the door on time, the number of discrete arguments the teen has with her sister. Counting behaviors provides objective data about progress—and if you (or your son or daughter) can turn it into a graph on an Excel spreadsheet, the feedback may be all the more powerful. *In fact, we have found that quite often graphs by themselves serve as an effective motivator without the need for any additional incentive.*

2. *Create a rating system to calculate improvement.* The simplest way to do this is to create a 5-point scale that you and your child might use independently to rate how things are going since the intervention was put in place. Here's what one might look like:

+2	A lot better
+1	Somewhat better
0	Same as before
−1	Somewhat worse
−2	A lot worse

Using this system, at the end of each day, you and your child could independently rate how successful the intervention was that day compared to the way things were before you started. Discuss any differences in your rankings, with each of you presenting data to support your ranking. See if you can reach an agreement; if not, split the difference. You should be shooting for +1 or +2 about 80% of the time and should periodically ask whether you've met the goal yet.

The idea of measuring progress may sound so burdensome that you are unwilling to take the project on. We would argue that people often give up on interventions or let them slide because they can't see that their effort makes any difference. Counting behaviors or using an informal rating scale counters this tendency to give up by giving both parents and kids a reason for continuing. Even small gains become visible, and those gains become motivators to continue the program.

Step 4: Create a Plan for Achieving the Goal

This may best be begun by considering the obstacles that are currently preventing your child from handling the problem situation successfully. Ask your teen what he sees as obstacles. If he can't think of any, you can bring up the things you have thought of. In the case of Jake, who is chronically late for school, he and his parents may identify obstacles such as staying up too late playing video games and sleeping through his alarm, not allowing enough time in the morning to do all that needs to be done before leaving the house, becoming distracted in the middle of getting ready for school, or leaving until morning things he could reasonably do the night before. The plan created should then outline how the obstacles will be addressed.

In the case of Maxine, a different approach might work. When youngsters have executive skills weaknesses that involve impulse control, emotional control, or flexibility, the approach we generally recommend is this:

- *Identify the triggers.* This means figuring out what immediately precedes the problem behavior that seems to set it off. In Maxine's case, it could be finding out her sister took something without asking, but it also could include her sister engaging in provocative behaviors designed to aggravate Maxine.

- *Establish the can't dos.* This means deciding what behavioral responses are off limits. In Maxine's case, reasonable *can't dos* might include yelling, swearing, or even physical aggression, if it comes to that.

- *List coping strategies or replacement behaviors.* What can Maxine do instead of blowing up? Identify two or three options, such as counting to 50 before saying anything, filling out a "complaint form" to be handed over to a parent, or walking around the block to cool down.

At each step (triggers, *can't dos*, coping strategies), you should give your teen the lead. Ask *her* what sets her off, ask *her* what she thinks the off-limits behaviors should be, and get *her* ideas for coping strategies or replacement behaviors. Of course you can offer suggestions, especially if your teen has trouble coming up with ideas, but the more your child has to offer, the better the plan is likely to be. On top of that, the thinking involved in coming up with the plan involves the very executive skills we're trying to build.

The same approach can be applied to situations in which youngsters react impulsively or inflexibly, as well as situations in which emotional control is lost (due to anger, frustration, or anxiety).

Step 5: Capture the Plan Succinctly in a Checklist or Reminder List

This becomes a sort of "cue card" to remind your child of the plan. Ideally, it should fit on a single sheet of paper (or, even better, an index card) and should look more like a brief checklist than a labor contract drawn up by a lawyer. An example of what Jake's checklist might look like appears on page 121. How Maxine's intervention can be depicted is shown on page 122.

Take Advantage of Technology

Whenever feasible, incorporate use of electronic media into the plan. Paper checklists, which can be posted in a prominent place as a reminder, are often invaluable, but smartphones and laptops can be programmed with alarms to serve as reminders, and this is where many teenagers live. Laptops also have "post-it" programs that can be posted to the desktop, acting as a reminder every time the user turns on the computer or shifts out of one screen to get to another.

Jake's Reminder List for Getting Ready for School on Time

The Night Before	
	Put all homework in backpack
	Put other things in backpack (e.g., gym clothes, permission slips, etc.)
	Get clothes ready for tomorrow
	Set alarm
	Lights off by 10:30
In the Morning	
	Get out of bed after no more than one "snooze alarm"
	Take 5-minute shower
	Get dressed
	Eat breakfast
	Brush teeth
	Ready for school by 6:30

Ask Your Child if He or She Wants Your Help

In developing the plan, you and your child should consider whether there's a role for you to play in carrying it out. Kids who hate being "nagged" are often willing to accept reminders if it's part of a plan they helped design. Jake, for instance, might ask his dad to check in on him at 10:00 P.M. to remind him he needs to start going through his list before lights out. When you agree to participate in the plan, write that down on the reminder list (for example, *To help me carry out this plan, my mom or dad will [or won't, depending on what follows]* _____).

Review the Plan One Last Time

When the plan is committed to paper, both you and your child should read it carefully to make sure it's what you both want. Is any part of the plan unclear or likely to be misinterpreted? Do you see any loopholes one of you might exploit as your child tries to follow the plan? Correct these problems before completing this step.

Step 6: Decide on a Trial Period

When the plan is completed and agreed on, decide how long you will try it out before revisiting it to make sure it's working. Of course, if something has been overlooked, changes can be made at any point, but we recommend you agree on a trial period before considering any substantive changes. A typical trial period might be 1–3 weeks, depending on the plan. The time span should be long enough to give it time to work but not so long that if it doesn't work your child digs a hole he can't get out of (for example, Jake is in danger of failing his first-period class because he's not following his plan).

Maxine's Plan for Controlling Her Temper

Triggers

- Sister borrowing my things without permission
- Sister making provocative comments to get me to react

Can't Dos

- Yell at sister
- Use ugly language

Coping Strategies/Replacement Behaviors

- Count to 50 before responding
- Fill out a "complaint form"
- Go for a walk around the block

Successes (one slash mark for each time I use the coping strategy successfully)

Step 7: Get the Plan Up and Running

The hardest part about this step is trusting the process to work—or trusting your child to follow the process. If you have a part in the plan (for example, providing cues or reminders), be sure to do what you said you were going to do *and no more*. For instance, if Jake's dad agrees to check in with him at 10:00 P.M., then he should check in with him just once (not again at 5-minute intervals thereafter). If this is hard for you, keep a log of how you think things are going to give yourself something to do while waiting for the trial period to end.

Step 8: Review the Plan and Revise If Necessary

You and your child may not agree about how well the plan is working. This is where having objective data and an agreed-on benchmark comes in handy. A record of tardiness from Jake's school should be easy enough to obtain, but Jake and his parents should also discuss how other elements of the plan have gone. Maybe Jake feels his parents are nagging him in the morning and that wasn't part of the agreement. Or maybe Jake's parents feel this is happening because he's hitting the snooze button two or three times, and he seems to be relying on them to harass him to get him out of bed. Try not to get too bogged down in details—especially if overall the plan is working—but you may need to alter it a little or add an addendum to further clarify roles or tasks.

Strategies to Use with Teens Who Resist the Teaching/Learning Process

If you're like many parents of the teens we work with, you read the previous section and muttered to yourself, *I wish!* Odds are your teen is one of the 75% who will need to be convinced or coaxed into this whole process because, as discussed in Chapter 2, your teen knows he has a problem but thinks he can manage it (but can't) or would like to handle it himself (he can't), or he doesn't believe he has a problem at all and brushes you off with a "Don't worry—if there's a problem, I'll handle it" (he won't). In all three cases, you will likely have to put your own specific goals for your child on the back burner and focus on your child's more immediate self-interest to get him to collaborate in this process.

It all starts with using something your child wants. You can either embed instructions for an executive skill into the process of the teen's attaining his goal or offer what the teen wants in exchange for his learning the skill you've identified as important. Let's say your son is eager to get his driver's license and buy a car. *Your* goal for him may be to get him planning for college, but that goal is not real enough to make him willing to make the effort. You can teach planning skills by helping him outline the steps he needs to go through to get his license and a car—skills that will be portable to other situations down the road, such as applying to colleges. We have presented these steps for driving under "Using Everyday Activities to Teach Executive Skills" later in the chapter.

Step 1: Identify a Goal Important to Your Teen

So the place to start is to talk with your teen about a goal that is important to him or her. Depending on your child's developmental stage (freshmen in high school are usually at a very different place than juniors and seniors, for instance), the goal may be short-term or longer-term, but whenever possible begin by talking about long-term goals. What does the teen want to do after finishing high school? Go to college? Get a job? Join the military? Move out of the house and into her own apartment? Move to a city and find a job, any job, so she can live on her own? Run away and join the circus? (Just kidding.)

Is the goal your child has selected one you can support or help with? Be specific about how you can help. If your child assumes, for instance, that you will pay for an apartment for him in Boston while he looks for a job for the summer before starting college and you're unable or unwilling to do that, let him know that now. Or if your daughter expects that once she gets her license you will buy her a car and you're thinking that once she gets her license you're willing to share your car with her, she needs to know that. If she still wants her own car, start talking about how to get a job to save the money she needs—and how fortuitous it is that the tasks involved in seeking and securing a job are filled with opportunities to grow executive skills! In any event, confirming or correcting assumptions can head off significant conflicts sparked by unspoken agendas.

Beginning with your teen's goal rather than your own may feel either frustrating or scary, especially if the gap in perception is wide. Focusing on a goal your child wants to work on doesn't mean you have to give up hope that he or she will set more long-term or "realistic" goals down the road, but if the gap between what you want for your teen and what your teen wants is wide, you may have little choice. If we had a magic formula for getting kids to see things with maturity and wisdom beyond their years, we would share it with you. Alas, we don't. With teens who don't share your viewpoint, your best bet is to go with a goal that matters to your teen and use it as an opportunity for teaching some skills that will be useful in the future. For example, your goal for your teen is that he maintain a B+ average in all classes. Your son's goal may be more like "as long as I'm not getting D's or F's." If that's what he's earning now, he will have to improve his executive skills just to bring his grades up to C—and if he pulls this off, he's learned something about setting and achieving goals. The next time, he may shoot for a more challenging goal, knowing he met the last one.

By all means, do not rain on your teen's parade at this point. Teens engaged in this process are new at this, and even though you may understand the complexity of the issues, laying out all the gory details may overwhelm them and make them feel less rather than more competent. The objective is not to demonstrate their immaturity, naïveté, or lack of knowledge of the "real world," even if that's what you want to do.

In the same vein, avoid pointing out how unrealistic your teen's expectations may be. For example, don't tell a teen who is applying for a highly sought-after job that she should spare herself the disappointment of not getting it and not apply. She'll need support and explanations after the fact, and those will be easier to provide if she doesn't fear hearing "I told you so." The "real world" is often a more effective teacher of difficult lessons than parents.

Avoiding Common Parental Traps

It's hard to avoid certain knee-jerk responses when you think your teen's decisions are setting him up for failure. You'd hardly be alone if you took the attitude "If he wants this badly enough, he can figure it out on his own. If he doesn't, it wasn't that important." This just doesn't apply for teens with significant executive skills weaknesses. They need help and monitoring to achieve their goals, and if you can provide it without taking over, you will have gone a long way toward helping your teen strengthen his skills. Another reaction to avoid is to say "Okay, if you want to do this on your own, go ahead—you'll find out how hard it is" or "Don't come crying to me when you can't figure it out." These statements convey that your objective is to maintain control and/or demonstrate your teen's inadequacy rather than boost skill development, and they can worsen conflict or communication problems between you and your child. The objective in all cases is to *provide just enough help or support for the teen to learn the skill.*

Step 2: Lay Out the Plan for Attaining the Goal

This is similar to Step 4 above, but since this goal is dear to your teen's heart, the teen should take the lead in outlining the plan. If she has no idea where to begin, list some possible options (for example, contacting the registry of motor vehicles to learn how to get a driver's license, signing up for driver's ed at school, or looking for driving schools online) and the basics of what she needs to consider, such as the cost of lessons, the time required, and how they will fit into her busy schedule. Again, embedding the teaching of executive skills within the plan for attaining a goal is covered for driving under "Using Everyday Activities to Teach Executive Skills," later in this chapter. But what if your teen's goal seems to offer little opportunity for executive skills development or you just can't get him motivated to work on a skill you believe is critical?

Joey was a 15-year-old we saw in our clinical practice. He was a very bright underachiever whose parents were concerned that his mediocre school performance was closing doors to the kinds of colleges he might get into if he lived up to his potential. His poor grades arose from his failure to hand in some homework assignments on time and his insufficient effort studying for tests, which led to poor test grades. His parents' goal for Joey was to have him manage his time better and to make better choices about how he was spending his time.

Unfortunately, this goal left Joey cold. So we, along with Joey's parents, had to get a little bit more creative to find a way to strengthen his executive skills. Joey was an avid skier who coveted an expensive pair of skis. As we worked with this family, it became evident that the skis were so desirable to Joey that he was willing to work on his parents' goal if that got him the skis. The plan we came up with ended up going beyond teaching just the executive skill embedded in the goal and taught Joey additional skills.

We worked out a system whereby Joey earned "points" (well, actually dollars, but to appear a little less mercenary, we often translate dollars into points for the incentive systems we devise) for grades of B– or better on tests and quizzes and for every week that he handed in all his homework on time. We planned it so that it would take much of the academic year for him to earn the skis (although we also arranged for the points to do "double duty" since they also translated into weekly spending money for Joey).

Saving money toward a long-term goal taught Joey response inhibition (or delayed gratification), an executive skill that's critical for learning money management. However, by tying it to academic performance, his parents were also able to get Joey to work on other executive skills that were not on his list of priorities. Because he had a goal he cared about, Joey was willing to spend time learning more effective study methods in order to bring his test grades up (we structured it so that the higher the test grade, the more points he earned). The incentive that mattered to him persuaded Joey not only to keep track of home-work assignments better, but also to plan his time more carefully and to spend time learning study strategies. His parents got what they were looking for, and Joey earned his skis.

Incentives that are attractive to teens can serve as a carrot to entice them to work on skills in keeping with parental goals. And as in the case of Joey, such a plan can produce additional benefits. But such plans need to be devised care-fully (and you may need to involve a third-party mediator to help negotiate this kind of plan) so that your teen is truly motivated to work on problem situations and executive skills that might otherwise hold no interest for him.

Using Everyday Activities to Teach Executive Skills

Have you ever thought about all the skills kids need to function independently as adults? (This is Peg talking:) When my then 19-year-old son got a job and an apartment on his own in Boston, he called me one night to find out how to make a chicken dish he really liked. When I talked with him later to find out how it had gone, he told me he had to throw the meal away because the chicken had gone bad—only then did I realize I'd never talked with him about food spoilage and expiration dates!

Even if you've already taught your teen executive skills via the other routes in this chapter, you and the teen may both gain extra confidence if you work on building skills within the everyday activities that are foundations for growing independence. We have found that this path to stronger executive skills is often neglected, so it might be worth your attention.

One way to identify routine activities to target is to look for the points at which your interests and your teen's intersect. Money management is an obvi-ous example: Your teen no doubt wants money to spend, and you no doubt want her to learn how to spend it responsibly. So strategies for learning responsible money management should serve the interests of both of you. Another possibil-ity is food. Kids have an interest in eating food that's appealing to them, and you have an interest in getting them to the point where they can budget, buy, and prepare food with the same level of skill you bring to these activities.

In Chapters 9–19 we'll look at each executive skill separately, showing you how you can use a variety of strategies, including skill instruction, to promote

the development of that skill. Here we'll look at the domains of everyday functioning instead, describing how certain routine activities tap certain executive
functions and how you can embed executive skills training into those areas of
functioning. Keep in mind, however, that these are just examples. Everyday life
is rich in opportunities to teach executive skills, and as you read through our
examples you may be able to think of additional ways you can use common
activities as a means to teach executive skills.

Driving

For teens, driving, perhaps more than any other activity, symbolizes independence and entry into adulthood. Because of this and because of the different
steps that can be part of the experience, driving represents an ideal vehicle for
addressing executive skills.

> *Executive Skills Involved*
>
> - Driver education
>
>   - Planning
>   - Task initiation
>   - Time management
>   - Flexibility
>   - Goal-directed persistence
>
> - Driving
>
>   - Sustained attention
>   - Response inhibition
>   - Emotional control
>   - Metacognition
>
> - Access to cars
>
>   - Time management
>   - Flexibility
>   - Emotional control
>
> - Car purchase
>
>   - Planning
>   - Task initiation

- Flexibility
- Goal-directed persistence
- Response inhibition

- Car maintenance/upkeep (repairs, inspection, registration)

  - Planning
  - Time management
  - Flexibility
  - Response inhibition
  - Emotional control

1. *Issues for teens.* Most teens will welcome the opportunity to drive. Issues are likely to arise around driving restrictions (time, car availability), car responsibilities, and car purchases if that is in the picture.

2. *Issues for parents.* For parents, the most significant concerns come in driving itself. As stated in Chapter 6, government and insurance statistics estimate more than 3,000 teens are killed yearly in car crashes and 350,000 are injured. Sixteen-year-old drivers are three times as likely as 17-year-olds and five times as likely as 18-year-olds to be involved in crashes. We will address the issue of safety below. Beyond safety there is the cost of driving (insurance, repairs, car purchase), which is in large part borne by parents, and ongoing negotiations about car availability.

3. *Steps in the process.* Unless you have a stronger investment than your teen in his or her getting a license, beginning with the driver education piece, let the teen take the primary role in making arrangements. This includes finding out who offers the course, comparative costs, starting and ending dates, and the schedule for classroom and road times. This must be coordinated with the teen's schedule to work around extracurricular commitments including jobs and participation in art, music, or sports activities. Parent schedules also need to be factored in for drop-off and pickup. As part of this process, have your teen speak with a representative from your insurance company or at least do it jointly so the teen can appreciate the cost and learn what he can do to decrease it (for example, discounts for good grades). Your level of support may range from simply telling the teen that he can start the process to cuing the teen to perform each step. Provide the least amount of help necessary for your teen to succeed.

Once your teen is ready to begin driving, safety is the prime consideration. We recommend the following steps. First, have your teen research teen driving contracts (available on the Internet) and sign one that you two can agree on. Second, have your teen investigate the most important safety features in cars so that she becomes educated about the various features and why they are important. Third, have your teen investigate whether crash prevention courses are available near you. These are hands-on, short driving courses that teach drivers how to best handle a car in an emergency situation. In New England, In Control (*www.driveincontrol.com*) offers such courses and has proven effective in reducing accidents; some insurance companies offer discounts for course completion. Fourth, since cell phone use while driving is a demonstrated cause of accidents, consider software such as iZup (*www.getizup.com*), which defers calls and text messages while the car is in motion.

Finally, you might have reason to believe that your teen will drive in a risky manner. For example, if your child has a history of risk taking involving speed and diminished awareness of danger (in bike riding, skateboarding, skiing, etc.), and/or a weakness in response inhibition, risky driving is likely. If your child has been diagnosed with ADHD, he is at greater risk for dangerous driving practices and automobile accidents. Or perhaps you've driven with your teen, and even when you're in the car, he does not drive safely. If so, there are a number of technologies that provide car data monitoring. As with the driving contract, if you decide to go down this road, have your teen investigate the options and suggest one that you can agree on. If you feel that it's more probable than not that your teen does not or will not drive safely, then we believe that while the monitoring system used may be open to negotiation, the choice of using a system is not. We respect the need for teen autonomy and trust, but given the accident statistics for teen drivers and the potential catastrophic results of an accident, we recommend erring on the side of safety.

You'll also have to decide when your teen will have access to cars and, if there is more than one car in the family, which one the teen will drive. In both cases safety should be the prime consideration. Your teen should always be driving the car with the best safety features if at all possible.

Preferably before starting to drive, your teen should also know and be able to demonstrate basic car maintenance (fluids, tire change), including how to read indicators and gauges. If possible, provide the teen with road service insurance and have her demonstrate how to use it.

If a car purchase is in the picture, communicate your limits—safety features, your contribution (if any), who will pay for repairs, what the cost of insurance will be, and who will pay what—before the search process begins. If safety is a prime concern, have the teen search for "safest cars for teens."

4. *Fading support.* Since issues with cars and driving generally persist as long as teens are living at home (and sometimes beyond that!), you will probably maintain some support, but if your teen has successfully (mostly) accomplished the above, he is well on his way to car independence. Fading support might include things like educating your teen about insurance in preparation for taking him off your policy. You might cease giving him reminders about car maintenance. Fading support might come in the form of allowing your teen to deal with traffic violations. Perhaps initially you make him go through the steps necessary to pay a parking ticket. Further down the road, he might be expected to deal with an insurance claim or violation with minimal assistance from you. Fading support is about easing your teen through the transition to independence, rather than expecting him to morph into a fully grown adult on his 18th birthday.

Money Management

Learning how to earn, save, and spend money is a key part of a teen's maturation process, and having money is a powerful source of independence. In our consumer-driven world, effective money management is a critical skill. Money management can be divided into three areas:

- *Earning and manipulating money:* Teens will typically accrue money through allowances, gifts (birthdays, holidays, etc.), and jobs. They need to know what to do with the money—cash, savings account, checking account, debit and credit cards.

- *Budgeting (their own and family finances):* Help your teen create her own budget (clothes, car maintenance, recreation) and involve her in the family budget (household expenses, etc.) if you are comfortable with the teen having that information and confident that it will not be posted on Facebook or some other public forum.

- *Shopping:* Your teen needs to know how to do comparison shopping and ways to save family money.

Executive Skills Involved

- Planning
- Organization

- Response inhibition
- Goal-directed persistence

1. *Issues for teens.* Getting teens involved in the money management process is not typically a problem since for most teens money is a powerful reinforcer and a source of independence. For teens involved in a variety of extracurricular activities (sports, music, drama), working throughout the school year may not be realistic. If this is true for your teen, you will need to decide whether you want to set allowances and budget on a schedule or as the need or demand arises. A teen who is working may expect full control of his own money and resist any parental intrusion. We encourage you to have your teen make some contribution to expenses directly related to his life (cell phones, car insurance, saving for college, clothes, etc.). This is especially important for teens who have difficulty with delayed gratification and are impulse buyers. As you will note below, we have built in some incentives for teens to be involved in money management through comparison shopping.

2. *Issues for parents.* You will have to decide what to provide for your teen in terms of money and other resources, and you'll have to do so over and over as your teen's needs and relative amount of freedom change. Teens often have a sense of entitlement about what they "deserve," and while attempts to set limits can lead to conflict, such limit setting is an important and ongoing part of the development process that continues into college and young adulthood.

3. *Steps in the process.* If an allowance is the source of money, you need to decide what you can afford and what, if any, responsibilities your teen will have to fulfill to earn the money. If your teen has a job, she will need to negotiate with you what her contributions to her own expenses will be.

How to manage money is an important part of this process. Will your teen use only cash, establish savings or checking accounts, or use debit and credit cards? If you have a local bank or credit union, you and your teen can meet with a bank representative to discuss various money management options. There are also a number of helpful websites (for example, CreditCards.com) that provide detailed information about various card options.

You can help your teen learn budgeting by handing out an allowance once a month rather than more frequently, but we recommend this only for teens who have demonstrated some ability to save. You can also show the teen what her specific expenses are in the context of family expenses (phone, car insurance, health insurance, food, clothes) and, by extension, what the family budget looks like.

Smart spending can be taught by having your teen comparison shop for desired items (phones, clothes, cars). You can extend this idea to big-ticket items for the family (TVs, computers, etc.): Tell the teen that if he does research that ends up saving the family money on such a purchase, you'll give him a percentage of the savings. You could do the same if your teen comes up with other ways to save the family money, such as reducing household electricity consumption.

4. *Fading support.* Whether your teen is living on an allowance or job income, fade support when she can stay within a mutually agreed-upon budget. An example of fading financial support might be paying out a teen's allowance in biweekly or monthly installments to allow him to allocate money himself.

Appointments

Appointments come into play in many areas of a teen's life: medical and dental checkups as well as visits for illness or injury; job interviews; regular car maintenance, repairs, and registration or inspection; and meetings with school staff. Teens need to decide, independently or jointly with you, what appointments need to be made when. The information must be remembered and stored, and the appointments completed.

Executive Skills Addressed

- Planning

- Task initiation

- Working memory

- Time management

1. *Issues for teens.* Your teen is probably used to a lot of help from you in making and keeping appointments. So he may view these responsibilities as an unwelcome chore or may just not have any idea how to go about this task.

2. *Issues for parents.* Teens who are learning this process need a safety net, because the consequences—as you know but they may not—can be costly to health or pocketbook if, for example, preventive dental care is neglected or car registrations are not renewed on time.

3. *Steps in the process.* As we recommended with chores, if possible, begin by having your teen set up and keep appointments that are relevant to her

needs. For students who are participating in sports, for example, having them schedule physicals is a good introduction to medical appointments. For teens who are driving, any appointment or scheduled event that relates to the availability of the car for them is a built-in motivation. This is also true for job interviews.

For other appointments, discuss with your teen why the appointment is important or necessary and walk the teen through the factors to consider: who needs to be called, what else is on the teen's schedule, and perhaps even an outline of what to say on the phone.

Early in this process, you may need to be close by to ensure that the teen records appointments made. The minute the phone is hung up or an e-mail is received, the date, time, and location of the appointment should be entered into the teen's primary scheduling device, which for most will be a cell phone. Your role as safety net is to record the appointments yourself as well as a backup.

You can also ensure that the teen uses an alarm or series of alarms. (This is Dick talking:) My son, who has particular trouble remembering appointments, will typically set two, or perhaps three, separate alarms for a single appointment. The first may sound a week in advance, the second a day or two in advance, and the third on the day of and a few hours prior to the appointment. Current cell phone technology and smartphones have made this process relatively easy, because multiple alarms can be set by voice command.

4. *Fading support.* You are likely to be involved in the appointment process for a fairly long period of time since you will anticipate issues that need to be addressed when your teen has not yet developed the same capacity. The goal, however, is for your teen to at least be able to follow through on the actual setup and completion of the appointment, even if you need to initiate the idea.

School Problems

Whether problems take the form of missing homework, chronic lateness to school or class, problems completing long-term papers and projects, or difficulty preparing for tests and exams, your teen's executive skills weaknesses are likely to manifest most obviously at school. It is in that environment where performance demands are unrelenting and all executive skills are called into play at one point or another. If and when school problems arise, it is important that both you and your teen have a plan in place to address them. In our experience, teens with executive skills weaknesses let small problems snowball into big ones more so than their peers. Hence, at the first sign of a problem, it is important to have a plan to address the issue.

Executive Skills Involved

- Depending on the nature of the problem, any one of the 11 executive skills, alone or in combination, may be involved.

1. *Issues for teens.* Students with significant executive skills issues are likely to have experienced some problems or failures at school by the time they reach high school and to feel that they have not lived up to the expectations of some adults. At a time when they want to be independent and manage their own lives, school problems confirm that they cannot manage on their own or perhaps live up to their expectations for themselves. These factors make it less likely that your teen will readily come to you to report a school problem.

2. *Issues for parents.* In the case of school problems, parents have to manage conflicting priorities. On the one hand, they have a legitimate interest in and a right to know about their child's school performance. On the other hand, if they keep managing the situation as they did in elementary or even middle school, the teen will miss out on the chance to develop the skills to address these problems more independently. At this stage in your child's life, you'll have to find a way to stay involved while inching your teen toward taking the lead in addressing problems with the teachers.

3. *Steps in the process.* Because your teen can dig herself into a hole that will be hard to get out of quickly, your priority should be to get timely information about school performance. Fortunately, schools and teachers have become increasingly reliable in providing up-to-date information through student portals about students' academic performance as well as upcoming homework, projects, and tests. We strongly encourage you to take advantage of these portals and, if your teen has a history of school difficulty, to talk to your teen both at the beginning of each school year and then periodically through the year about how she will address problems that arise. Emphasize that you prefer your teen to take the lead in resolving a problem by meeting with a teacher or school counselor and coming up with a plan. This gives the teen an opportunity for independence, personal responsibility, and development of the notion of professional relationships, which she will need in college and/or in a job.

Laying this groundwork means that whenever you notice via a portal that your teen's performance has declined, you can ask your teen if he has met with the teacher. If not, encourage your teen to do so and discuss how you will know the problem has been resolved. Ask for a specific timeline from the student, as in "Within 2 days, I will have met/called/e-mailed X, explained my situation, and discussed a plan for how to resolve it." Then you can check with the teen to see if he has followed through on the plan. Obviously, the teen can say he has when in fact he hasn't. While the information you get through the portal won't be immediate, if the problem is specific and involves late or missing assignments, test grades, or a missing project, using the portal will give you an independent source of information. If you have reason to doubt that your teen has attempted to resolve the problem at all, e-mailing the school staff is the next logical step, and then independent verification by e-mail to the teacher should be part of the plan going forward.

   4. *Fading support.* Through high school and perhaps into college, depending on the nature and extent of school problems, parents should continue to monitor school performance and, when problems arise, at least check to see whether the teen has followed through on the plan. School performance in high school and in college, if parents are responsible for tuition, should involve ongoing monitoring for students with executive skills weaknesses. The transition to college, for these teens, carries a fairly significant risk since the supports that have been in place are no longer available. Tuition is not the only consideration here. Failure to successfully complete freshman year has significant psychological consequences for the teen and parents. Considering this as well as the cost of college, we believe that parents have a legitimate role in monitoring their teen's success.

Chores

For teens and parents, chores—vacuum the floor, wash the dishes, empty the dishwasher, do the laundry, feed the pets, shop for groceries—are often a contentious issue. Yet, as adults, if we hadn't developed these skills and made them part of our daily routine, we'd be wearing dirty clothes, eating out regularly, and living in a pigpen.

Executive Skills Involved

- Task initiation
- Planning/prioritization
- Organization

- Time management

- Goal-directed persistence

- Sustained attention

1. *Issues for teens.* If you are just starting to expect your child to do chores now, anticipate resistance. To decrease this resistance, start with chores that are relevant to the teen's life and that she will need to do as an adult (washing clothes, shopping for and cooking a meal for friends or family, taking care of pets, car repairs, cleaning the bathroom, etc.). Also work up from those that require the least effort to those that require the most. On a scale of 1 to 10 (1 representing the least effort and 10 the most), have the teen rate the effort involved in each chore and then start with the chores rated least effortful. Try to find chores that capitalize on your teen's independence, such as driving siblings, dropping parents off at appointments, or cooking a meal for friends. If you still get significant resistance, tie chores to allowance or to privileges such as driving. If possible, make some of the chores part of a family routine and set aside time to do them together. Alternatively, establish a time frame for the chore and let the teen pick the time to do it as long as it is finished by the deadline.

2. *Issues for parents.* Typical issues that arise around chores include conflict over uncompleted chores or chores not done to the parents' satisfaction. Parents need to negotiate with teens what will happen if the teen doesn't follow through on the commitment to complete a chore. As we mentioned in Chapter 5, the best arrangement is a "first–then" system, where teens can pursue their plans after chores are completed. Typically teens will be more likely to complete chores if failure to complete them leads to decrease of independence and loss of free time.

3. *Steps in the process.* Start with tasks that are most relevant to your teen's life and future independence and enlist the teen's help in a way that is a genuine contribution to the family. Reward efforts with praise and, if necessary, privileges and tangible items (cash, clothes, etc.). Remember that learning to do chores is a gradual process for teens and that you and the teen are likely to have different ideas about how to do some things. As long as your teen is moving toward completing the task and aiming for your standard, he is making progress.

4. *Fading support.* When teens are completing agreed-upon chores with only very occasional reminders and when they are given a new chore to do and complete it without nagging, you can fade active and ongoing monitoring.

Getting Ready in the Morning

Why is it so aggravating to have to remind your teen to allow time to eat a good breakfast, to watch your teen waste time going back upstairs to fetch forgotten items for his backpack three or four times, and to see him rush out without hat or gloves even though the temperature is 20 degrees? Because we all know that by the time children reach adolescence, they've been through this drill a million times. And the fact is that most of the time they do know what's required—what time to get up, what they need to do to get ready, what they need to take to school. Unfortunately, there is a disconnect in the brain of almost all teens between knowing and doing—executive skills deficits or no deficits. And if we could go back, we'd remember that it took us a while to stick to our own schedule religiously, and we probably still slip up sometimes. We also know, however, that getting out of bed and getting ready in a timely fashion on a regular basis is critical to high school and college as well as job performance. So if your teen consistently has trouble in this area, this is an important skill to work on.

Executive Skills Involved

- Planning

- Organization

- Task initiation

- Time management

- Goal-directed persistence

1. *Issues for teens.* Initiating the wake-up and morning routine involves a number of potential barriers for teens. During adolescence, biological and social factors contribute to changes in sleep patterns. The result is that teens' "sleep clock" shifts forward so that they are awake later at night. Unfortunately, few school systems accommodate this change. The result is that teens are going to bed later but waking up early, and hence are somewhat sleep deprived, tired on waking, and often cranky. School is not necessarily a preferred activity, so the incentive to get up is diminished, and if they are not prepared or are having problems at school, there is an additional disincentive. There is also the fact that teens will overestimate the amount of time they actually have to get ready in the morning and underestimate the actual amount of time the process will take. A separate but complicating factor relates to the fact that sleep deprivation will degrade certain types of executive skills, such as working memory and sustained attention, and these are important for school functioning.

2. *Issues for parents.* For single- or two-parent families with working parents and/or other children to get ready, morning in general can be a stressful time. With a teen, particularly one who has had wake-up or morning routine difficulties, the stress is magnified. Parents will be concerned about how their own routines may be disrupted if the teen is late, and conflicts about getting up and getting ready in a timely fashion are routine.

3. *Steps in the process.* The first step in the process is for your teen to manage his own wake-up. This requires an alarm of the teen's choosing and, at least in the early stages, some sort of backup plan for what you should do if the teen is not awake by a certain time. Part of the success at this stage depends on finding an approach that suits your teen's personality. Some teens like to set an alarm early and go through multiple snooze alarms. Some teens will get up earlier if the first activity in their routine is one of their choice. That might be listening to particular music, watching a favorite TV show, or checking Facebook.

As a parent, your concern is that the teen get up and out in a way that allows him to get to school on time. If the teen wakes up on time but meanders through his routines and is late as a result, you can ask him for possible solutions to the problem once you have some data, such as the number of times the school has reported the child tardy. Most schools impose consequences for routine lateness, and parents can utilize this if it happens in a fashion timely enough to have an impact on the teen's behavior.

Incentives are another way to help your teen get through the morning routine. Offer the teen money for breakfast out after a certain number of days of on-time arrival at school. If your child has "auto envy" and is a decent driver, offer her the opportunity to periodically drive the preferred car (as long as it's a safe car). If your teen routinely forgets items that she will need throughout the day and you have school feedback about that, or if your teen is in the habit of calling you to drop items off, ask if she would be willing to put everything in one place the night before or create a checklist she can review to ensure that materials have been packed. If your teen repeatedly forgets items, giving some sort of cue, including asking her if she has everything prior to leaving, is a step toward handing this off to the teen over time.

4. *Fading support.* The markers for fading support with wake-up and morning routines are pretty concrete. When your teen is able to get herself out the door with only a few late episodes per semester and is not calling you more than once every 6 to 8 weeks for a forgotten item, the skill is fairly well learned. Specifically, this would mean going from daily checks that she is up to twice-weekly checks to no checks as long as she makes an appearance by a certain time or has no more than two late notices from school in a term.

We have not tried to address all the areas or skills that teens will need to have some mastery of in order to live independently. If you wonder where your teen rates in terms of adult living skills or have concerns about the skills he should be working on, we recommend that you look at the Casey Life Skills assessments (*www.caseylifeskills.org*). These assessments, which can be completed by parents and teens, provide ratings of life skills in a range of different areas (for example, communication, money management, social relationships, self-care, work and study skills) that are essential for independent adult living. In addition, this website provides a variety of resources to parents and teens for addressing and mastering these life skill areas. The assessment is free, and we have found it to be very valuable in our work with parents and teens. We encourage you to use it as a resource.

Part III

PUTTING IT ALL TOGETHER

8

···

Advance Organizer

In Chapter 7 we laid out the steps for teaching an executive skill to your teen, with particular emphasis on creative ways to enlist the participation of the 75% of teens who believe they either don't have a problem or don't need adult help or guidance to address it. Our focus in Chapter 7 was on the teen's growing independence. Since the teen wants increasing autonomy and you want your teen to become an effectively independent adult, this should be the central theme in your plans to teach your teen an executive skill. It involves allowing your teen to take the lead as much as possible. You will need to use the teen's personal goals as an incentive and make the effort to build executive skills within the activities that are critical to independence, from driving to money management, in addition to the ongoing functions you may have been struggling with since your teen was much younger—school problems, chores, and getting ready for the day.

In the 11 chapters following this one, you'll have a chance to design your own plans for building specific executive skills that you now know are a big issue for your teen. In each of those chapters you'll do a more detailed assessment of your child's ability to use an individual skill and then get tips for building that skill in everyday activities. We give you a detailed illustration in each chapter and also answer some questions parents often ask.

Before you get started on the individual skills covered in the rest of Part III, this chapter provides a set of strategies that will help you decide how and where to begin.

1. Provide the Minimum Help Necessary for Your Teen to Be Successful

The preceding chapters have offered a variety of ideas for what you *can* do to help your teen build executive skills. But how much *should* you do? When dealing with teens, less is often more. You are both seeking the same outcome: having your teen become the problem solver and decision maker. In most cases, the teen will naturally resist your help, and you want to minimize the chance that the teen will become or remain dependent on you, so it's up to you to figure out how much help is truly necessary and how much would only instill increased dependence. Here are some guidelines:

• *If a simple environmental modification will work, use it.* A voicemail, note, or text message reminding your son to empty the dishwasher before he goes to the dance may take care of the problem. In the case of regular chores or routines, you can try the reminders for a few weeks, tell him that you are going to stop them, and see if he continues to do the chore. If not, return to the reminders.

• *Whenever possible, communicate indirectly (for example, note, text message).* The idea is to create distance between you and your teen so that the cue can work without the two of you being in the same space at the same time.

• *If cues continue to be necessary, ask your teen to develop her own cues.* This is a way to hand off the skill to the teen so that reminders occur by her choice and in her words.

• *Whenever possible, try to avoid personally reminding your teen, especially in a repetitive fashion.* Parents often talk too much, include lessons, lectures, and nagging and use an irritated tone of voice when it comes to reminders. More often than not, this leads to conflict.

• *Whenever possible, if your teen requires more instruction or direction to learn a skill, use an outside expert rather than yourself to provide the direction.* Ultimately, if teens are going to be independent problem solvers, they need to use the people and information available in their environment rather than parents as problem solvers. While we all may feel good that from time to time our children ask us for help, this does not benefit their executive skills in the long run, unless our information is clearly instructional and over time they internalize the information and stop coming to us.

2. Identify One Executive Skills Weakness and the Specific Situations Where the Weakness Is Manifested

• *Give your teen the choice of what situation to work on first, or if the problem involves only one specific issue (for example, getting up and going in the morning), the option of how to address it.* This is a continuation of what we have suggested all along—anything that increases the teen's interest in both the problem and the solution enhances the teen's investment and the likelihood of mastery and control.

• *If your teen is open to help, choose a situation where implementation can be shared.* By making yourself available and letting your teen decide in what way you can provide help, you decrease the burden the task places on you. The objective is to fade your help over time, but not so quickly that your teen fails. If this model works for one problem or situation, this opens the door for using it in other situations.

• *Start with a problem that is small and easily tackled, if possible.* This is confidence building for you and your teen and increases the likelihood that the teen will be willing to work on other problems. With the morning routine, for example, if you can move from waking your teen to having her wake herself, this is a great beginning on this important multistep daily activity, and it eliminates what can be a source of aggravation for both of you.

• *Start with a problem whose resolution would lead to your teen's life and your own going more smoothly.* The morning routine is a good example because it is a typical source of stress for both teens and parents. *Not* starting out on a bad foot can change the entire tone of the rest of the day.

3. In Deciding What Skill and Situation to Address, Evaluate the Imprint the Problem Has on Your Teen's and Your Life

• *If a particular skill weakness puts your teen at immediate risk, address that executive skill first.* This is the place where parental judgment and decision making override teen choice. For example, if your teen has weaknesses in response inhibition or sustained attention, which you fear pose a risk of unsafe driving or substance use, address these situations first. Typically, this means closer monitoring of behavior and what will strike teens as parental intrusiveness. As we said earlier, a parent's fundamental job is to keep the teen "in the game." This does not mean that parents lock up their teens for the duration of adolescence, but it does mean that parents look for ways to balance choice and risk management.

• *Also make problems that could narrow the teen's options for the future a priority.* Academics and behavior in school are the most obvious examples. If your teen's executive skills weaknesses lead to academic underperformance or failure or disciplinary issues in school, address these situations first because they have both immediate and long-term implications.

• *If you are not dealing with immediate or future risk, but rather a lack of self-reliance, the place to begin is with everyday activities.* As recommended in Chapter 7, you can use the Casey Life Skills assessments to identify life domains that are a problem for your teen. Also in Chapter 7, we've listed the steps to teaching executive skills that lead to successful money management, responsible driving, independent handling of appointments, and other areas of functioning. The advantage of working in these areas is that they involve a range of executive skills, all of which will be useful and ultimately necessary for your teen to master, and which at the same time reduce their reliance or dependence on you.

• *The easiest activities to start with are those that are likely to accord with your teen's desires, such as driving and money management, but any one of them should be fair game to address.*

• *Always take advantage of some objective or goal your teen is invested in as a method for teaching executive skills.* Since virtually any goal requires planning, time management, sustained attention, task initiation, goal-directed persistence, and metacognition, personal goals that are a high priority for your teen are ideal vehicles for learning these executive skills and have the added advantage of built-in motivation if they come from your teen.

4. Be Positive and Flexible as You Work Through the Plan

• *Involve your teen in developing and implementing the plan.* We do not want to sound like a broken record, but if the plan comes entirely from you, it fails on two levels: your teen remains dependent on you, and your teen is likely to have reduced investment in the success of the plan.

• *If you are working together with your teen, remember the importance of goodness of fit.* What you think might be a good idea or what works for you may not work for your teen, particularly if in your self-assessment (see Chapter 3) you found that your strengths and weaknesses are different from those of your teen.

• *Expect to have to tweak your strategies.* Learning these skills is a work-in-progress for teens, and they are changing and adapting as they develop.

• *Provide liberal praise and positive feedback.* Although it may not always seem to be the case, teens value the positive recognition of their parents, and this is a good way for parents to help teens recognize and remember these skills for future use.

5. Meet Resistance with Creativity

If your teen refuses to work on any executive skills, don't throw up your hands—be prepared.

• *Negotiate.* If you have approached this situation with your teen as a "have to" or a "do it or else," consider offering an exchange: you'll give up something you want if the teen will give up something she wants (or do something you want). For example, if you want chores around the house done in exchange for use of the car, change the chores to errands you need done and offer the car if she'll run a couple of errands before she goes off with her friends. Or if you've said no video games until all of your teen's homework is done, negotiate a certain amount of homework for a certain amount of game time.

• *Consider more powerful reinforcers.* In our experience, parents are often cheap in terms of what they will offer, in part because they are annoyed at having to offer anything in the first place. If you accept that these are difficult skills for your teen, understand that it is going to take a good reason for the teen to make the effort.

• *If your teen still refuses to work on the skill, build in logical or natural consequences.* In Chapter 5, we reviewed the use of privileges in designing "first–then" contingencies whereby the teen gains access to what she wants only after doing some of what you want.

• *If these approaches do not work and the problems persist, consider outside help, such as a coach.* We have presented a detailed description of coaching in Chapter 20.

9

....

Enhancing Response Inhibition

Response inhibition is the capacity to think before you act—to resist the urge to do or say something before you've had a chance to evaluate the situation and the possible consequences. In adolescence, response inhibition is the most critical of executive skills. Weakness in response inhibition may be the executive skills deficit most likely to cause parents of adolescents to lose sleep. You may have seen signs of your child lacking this skill ever since infancy—the child couldn't seem to resist going after what he wanted, he was the first kid to take a risk when something looked like fun, or maybe he was quick to mouth off or hit when angered or even irritated. But now, for the first time, not only does your teen desperately want independence and the freedom to make his own decisions; he also has the means and opportunity to go for it. Perhaps you kept a tight rein on your son when he was younger, to protect him from himself. But now you don't have the power or the proximity to do that, and worrying about whether your teen's impulses will lead him to catastrophic risk causes you constant worry.

How Response Inhibition Develops

Response inhibition emerges first in infancy. In its most basic form, having response inhibition allows an infant to "choose" to respond or not respond to a situation, person, or object. Prior to the development of response inhibition, the infant is more passive, more at the mercy of what comes into his world, but once the infant is able to combine the ability to respond or not respond with the ability to move by crawling or walking, we see the earliest evidence of

149

self-regulation of behavior. Now the infant or toddler can "decide" to move or not move or, over a long period of time, to engage or not engage in a particular behavior. As children develop language, they also develop the ability to inhibit their responses because they can internalize rules set by adults (for example, "Don't touch the outlet").

In the development of executive skills, response inhibition plays a fundamental role because it enables the other executive skills to develop. A child or adolescent at the mercy of her impulses cannot initiate, sustain attention, manage time, plan, or organize in an effective way. If your teen has weak response inhibition, you may have observed that she seems scattered in many areas of life. In contrast, the teen who has the capacity to think before she acts and appreciate the consequences of her actions not only gains the ability to get things done but also is in a better position to make good decisions.

As they are growing, children typically become more adept at using most executive skills. However, response inhibition does not develop so steadily. According to neuroscience research, this executive skill may be more vulnerable to disruption in adolescence. Scientists studying how the brain changes during the teen years report that there is something of a "disconnect" between those centers of the brain where emotions and impulses are processed and the prefrontal cortex, where thinking before acting, or rational decision making, happens. We now know that over the course of adolescence and into adulthood these connections become stronger and faster through a process of pruning and myelination, described in Chapter 1. These strong connections make it possible for young people to temper their emotions and impulses with reason, but until those connections are firmly in place, teens are more prone to make decisions rashly, under the influence of peers, and based on "gut feelings," without the inhibition and judgment that the frontal lobes can provide.

To make matters worse, the adolescent shift toward greater influence by peers and challenging of parental authority contributes to impulsivity. Teenagers typically engage in what we defined earlier as context-dependent behavior, meaning basically that they get wrapped up in the moment. When with peers, they're more likely to go with the flow of their friends than to think about the consequences of a behavior that seems so appealing right now. Likewise, when they are involved in any situation or activity they find immediately pleasurable (video games, social media, driving fast, alcohol, sexual activity), that pleasurable activity is likely to rule their immediate behavior. And with the decreased controls on them exerted by society as a whole, they have increasing freedom to make poor decisions. As parents, you don't want to clamp down on your teens as if they're still 8 years old, because that would be a hindrance to the natural and necessary process of building independence. So the challenge is to establish enough controls to ensure that bad decisions result in good lessons learned and not danger or permanent damage to them or others.

How does your teen's ability to control impulses stack up against what is developmentally appropriate? The questionnaire on page 152 can help you further clarify the answer to this question, either con-

> *Risks are increased with both friends and an audience.*
> —Ben, age 17

firming or denying your initial assessment from Chapter 2, by looking a little more closely at response inhibition. Feel free to photocopy it if you want to use the form more than once, such as for another teen.

Building Response Inhibition

If your answers to the questions in the questionnaire suggest that your teen struggles with response inhibition, the following guidelines are important.

• *Assume that in the presence of peers your teen will have reduced impulse control.* In some situations, such as school, this issue is less critical, since there should be other adults to monitor and set expectations and limits. Open-ended social situations are the real areas of concern. First, make sure that prior to the time your teen is going out the door you have established clear expectations, limits, and consequences. We reviewed these in some detail in Chapter 6, but essentially this means knowing where your teen is going, whom the teen will be with, and what time the teen will return home. You also should have in place a procedure for how and when your teen will tell you about a change in plans. If you are expecting adults to be on hand to supervise house parties or sleepovers, talk to those adults ahead of time and ensure that your teen will stay on the premises for the planned duration of the party unless you're notified otherwise. Yes, your teen will object to this "surveillance." If you feel yourself wavering in the face of this opposition, all you need to do is read the police reports routinely published in newspapers about events that unfold at unsupervised parties.

• *Expect your teen to choose fun activities over challenging or nonpleasurable ones.* If the unappealing tasks have deadlines, such as for school projects, college applications, or even chores, you will need to check to see if they're being completed or if there are consequences for failure to complete them. You also

How Well Does Your Teen Inhibit Impulses?

For each item in the chart, first decide whether the statement to the left or right of *BUT* describes your teen better. Then rate the degree to which that statement applies to your teen. The number of items for which you chose the right-hand statement is an indicator of how much improvement your teen may need in the skill overall. Your ratings indicate possible targets for skill building: Where you chose "pretty much" or "very much" for a left-hand statement, your teen is demonstrating good use of the skill in that particular domain. "Pretty much" or "very much" for right-hand statements indicates areas that may need the most work.

Just a little	Pretty much	Very much				Just a little	Pretty much	Very much
			Some kids think about what might happen before they act.	BUT	Other kids act without thinking.			
			Some kids keep quiet or raise their hand to speak in class.	BUT	Other kids get in trouble for talking too much in class.			
			Some kids think about the consequences before they do something.	BUT	Other kids just act. They don't waste time thinking about the consequences.			
			Some kids take their time before making up their mind.	BUT	Other kids just "go with their gut."			
			Some kids think about how others will react when they say something.	BUT	Others kids say what's on their mind without worrying what effect it has on others.			
			Some kids are able to walk away from confrontation or provocation by a peer.	BUT	Other kids react immediately and challenge the peer.			
			Some kids can say no to a fun activity if other plans are already made.	BUT	Other kids go with the fun activity immediately in front of them.			

From *Smart but Scattered Teens*. Copyright 2013 by The Guilford Press.

may need to help your teen by discussing ways to control or eliminate distractions.

- *To help your teen delay gratification, use waiting periods for things she wants to do or have.* Learning to wait is the foundation for response inhibition and is a skill that teens need to develop. "First–then" schedules accomplish this goal ("*First* do your homework; *then* you can use the computer, take the car, etc.").

- *Require your teen to earn some of the things he wants as another way to teach delayed gratification and response inhibition.* Having your teen save for part of driver education, car insurance, or a cell phone, helps to combat the expectation that "I want it and deserve it right now."

- *Prepare your teen for situations that require impulse control by regularly reviewing the rules in advance.* This would include activities such as prohibition of cell phone use while driving, the use of seat belts, letting you know about changes in plans, and expectations about acceptable and unacceptable behaviors.

- *Immediately before your teen goes into a situation that may test response inhibition, review a few specific rules again.* When you do this, your teen might listen more carefully if you present these rules in the context of your caring about her and wanting her to be safe.

The Road as Racetrack: Managing Driving Speed

Bella loved to drive. More than that, Bella loved to drive *fast*. Having recently turned 16, she didn't yet own a car. But on Saturdays, when the weather was nice, her mother would let her borrow her blue coupe for local errands and to visit friends. Their house was on a rural back road that wound 6 miles in a gentle decline, ending at the limit of the small town where Bella would go to the movies or the comic book store.

This road was Bella's racetrack. She loved to push the coupe into a tightly wound corner and feel the tug on her body. She imagined herself completing this or that turn along the edge of the Grand Canyon, kicking rocks and red dust out into the abyss. The yellow 20-mile-per-hour signs and sharp curve warning arrows had her scared at first, but now she knew every twist and looked forward each time to having the road pass under her faster than before.

"Mom, can I borrow your car?"

It was a sunny Saturday in April, and Bella was poking her mother gently in the back as she stooped and planted bulbs in the driveway garden beds.

"Umm, sure Bella . . . be careful, though. The roads are still wet. The keys are in the dash."

She reached her arm around in front of her mother's face and jingled the keys, then took off up the driveway toward the garage.

"Buckle your seat belt, Bella!"

She brandished her trowel as Bella rolled by. Bella waved and gave her a thumbs-up in the rear window, then turned out into the road. The road was wet, but the sun was out, and even as Bella started to drive, she thought the road looked like a photo negative, with puddles of drying gray spreading out against the damp asphalt. It was warm, so she put the sunroof and the windows down and cranked up the radio. She hit a set of turns and leaned on the gas pedal, cranking the wheel back and forth with one hand and hunching slightly forward in concentration.

In the middle of the drive, there was a lull in the grade that opened out to almost a quarter of a mile of straightaway before a series of switchbacks brought you down to the base of the hill. Here the double yellow line turned dotted on one side, and Bella stepped on the gas, crossing over and blowing by a sedan in front of her. She lingered on the wrong side of the road for a moment, watching the car shrink in her rearview mirror. She pulled back into her lane just as both lines went solid and prepped for a sharp left-hand turn that followed the straightaway. In doing this, she looked out the lower left corner of the windshield, and so failed to see the police cruiser wedged into a slight dimple in the trees that lined the right side of the road.

After the officer gave her a ticket, Bella turned around. Speeding—54 in a 30—and a warning for reckless operation. Reckless operation? Bella thought she was in complete control the whole time. Nevertheless, she felt tense and confused and headed home because she did not know what else to do. She would have to tell her parents, she knew, both because she lacked the money to pay the ticket and because if they found out about it months later from a hike in their insurance premiums, the punishment would be compounded.

Bella walked into the house and saw her mom and dad sitting at the kitchen table with the newspaper split between them.

"Hey, guys."

"Hey there, I thought you were going downtown." They glanced at her and smiled, then returned to reading.

"Yeah, well, I was. I planned to. But I kind of ran into a little bit of a problem."

"Mmm. What kind of little bit of a problem?" Each turned a page.

"Well, I was driving downtown, and I got pulled over. And I . . . "

"Pulled over? By the police? Bella! Please tell me we are talking about a broken headlight."

Bella walked over to the table where her parents now sat erect. She sat down, took the ticket from her pocket, unfolded it, and slid it gently across the table onto the newspapers in front of them. Both of her parents were silent as they read it, and when they finished, they looked at her for a few seconds; finally, her father spoke.

"Bella, as you can probably understand, your mom and I are worried and angry about this. It reflects a neglect of the law and a compromise of our trust. We pay your insurance and let you use the car under the assumption that you do so responsibly and safely. In effect, you lied to us."

"I didn't lie! It wasn't like I meant to do this. You guys told me you thought I was a good driver. I get it, but I don't think it's that big a deal."

"Twenty-four miles over the limit was never something we expected, Bella," her mother said. "And you don't think of it as a big deal because you haven't experienced the consequences of something like this before."

Her father continued. "Bella, we've talked before about what we would do if we encountered this with you. This was dangerous and foolhardy on your part; you acted like a kid in an adult environment, and it came back to bite you. Fortunately or not, the adult world has its own consequences, and first and foremost you will address these on your own."

"Which means what?"

"You are going to pay for the ticket," her mother said. "You can get a job or work around the house and we will pay you. States vary in penalties for teens, but it is likely that most states will take your license away for a month or two. They will also put points on your license, which will make you susceptible to much higher future penalties, unless you take a course in defensive driving. You will pay for this course. You will also pay a portion of the increase in your insurance premiums."

> It's important for the parents to drive with the kid before allowing her in the car alone again.
> —Ben, age 17

"What about me getting a car? Two months ago we agreed it was time to start keeping an eye out for a car for me."

Her mother chuckled and continued. "Yes, I know we had talked about that in the past. For the time being, you won't be able to drive, so it won't be an issue. In the future, though, if we consider it, we would want to install a device that would monitor your speed and periodically check it to make sure you are driving responsibly. For now we'll need to do that in my car. Understand, Bella, this isn't a conflict between you and us. This is us helping you confront the problem now and avoid it in the future."

> *Once a teen goes fast once, she'll absolutely do it again. So Bella's parents do need to monitor her driving.*
> —Teo, age 15

> *What the parents decided on does accomplish the goals, but I would say the parents should not let Bella alone until she can prove that she can be responsible.*
> —Lorie, age 16

Bella spent many hours in her mother's garden beds. She earned the money and reapplied for her license.

> *Most teens will not be this compliant with punishment.*
> —Tasha, age 17

Q & A

Okay, Bella is a bad driver. What exactly does that have to do with her executive functions?

Bad drivers come in many different flavors. Some don't pay attention, some have poor vision, some are driving unfamiliar vehicles, some are just not very coordinated. Bella is an uninhibited driver, a whole different kind of problem. She isn't a bad driver because she can't pay attention or is physically impaired. Instead, her poor impulse control leads her to perform dangerous maneuvers that put her and other drivers at risk. Response inhibition is an important executive skill because it serves as risk management system, instantly conducting a risk–benefit analysis of almost every decision we make, even when we don't think about it explicitly. Risk is everywhere, and some risk taking is good. Without it people wouldn't reach their full potential. But when a person with a faulty mental "risk calculator" is behind the wheel of a car, she is liable to do things that are extremely unsafe. It's also worth noting that Bella's recklessness is due in part to her age; it's no coincidence that her demographic has the highest insurance rates. She most likely isn't aware firsthand of what can happen when a driver loses control. Naïveté combined with an appetite for risk is dangerous but not unmanageable.

Our teen has a problem with response inhibition, but it isn't related to driving. She has always been a class clown. It's extremely difficult for her to curb in-class outbursts, not only because she has poor response inhibition, but also because she believes that her reputation among her peers depends on this "performance." She isn't purposefully rude; she says she "just can't help it." What can we do?

This is a fairly common situation for parents of bright young teens who have difficulty with response inhibition. Not only are the outbursts disruptive for the class, but teens who play this role are constantly interrupting their own thought processes with tangential ideas. Sometimes this is a positive attribute; these teens are often outside-the-box thinkers, adept at free association and unique problem solving. But when it manifests as class clowning, whether out of boredom or socially driven, it's counterproductive. Some of the other techniques we describe in this book, like writing down keywords or following an outline, might help mitigate this problem by keeping your teen focused, essentially distracting her from distractions. If the problem is systemic, coordinating special seating arrangements with teachers might help. Sitting in front near the teacher also puts the rest of the class out of a student's line of sight, removing some of the visual incentives for her to try to entertain an audience. There also might be some merit in simply encouraging your teen to incorporate her natural sense of humor into productive responses. Witticisms and jokes don't have to be antagonistic; a valuable answer, accompanied by a playful quip, might garner admiration from both peers and teachers. Obviously your teen prizes her sense of humor. Sometimes the solution is more about channeling it effectively than trying to suppress it.

So how do we mediate reckless driving? What if our teen is doing this, but we only know about it through hearsay or our own suspicions, not a traffic ticket?

True, Bella's case is easier to diagnose and deal with because she got caught. Violating the law has its own consequences, often more serious ones than you would otherwise hand down yourself. As evident from the statistics cited earlier, driving poses risks, and the danger increases significantly for a teen with impulse control problems. What should you do? Put your teen in a safe car. An Internet search for "safe cars for teens" will provide you with a range of options. Consider a defensive driving or crash prevention course if one is available in your area. Consider an in-car driver-monitoring system. While this may seem extreme, if your teen has a history of impulsive behavior and risk taking, you

> I would also make education an important key point. Teenagers who had been exposed to the dangers of poor driving in a way that could not be ignored would be more likely to factor it into their judgment. I would also suggest that the parents make clear what their own consequences will be for tickets.
>
> —Tasha, age 17

need to know that he doesn't represent a risk to himself or others. If you chose not to use such a system before you had "proof," once you do have evidence of dangerous driving, it should be a condition of driving again. As your teen gets older and gains driving experience and his frontal lobes mature, he probably will not need the system over the long term. If your teen is willing to wait before getting a license, let him. Driving risk decreases with age.

10

....

Strengthening Working Memory

Working memory involves two different but related skills. The first is the ability to hold information in mind while performing complex tasks. At a relatively simple level, one example would be holding in mind the prices of three items while we add them up to see if we can afford to buy them all. Another simple example is holding in mind a question we've been asked as we search for and formulate an answer. A related but more complex aspect of working memory gives us the ability to draw on past learning or experience and apply it to the situation at hand or predict future outcomes. We can see a glimpse of this in the arithmetic problem or in the question from somebody. Both of those depend on some past learning or experience that would bear on the question or problem. However, in the more complex aspect of working memory, we can look at ourselves in a current situation, reach back into our experience to see ourselves in similar past situations, and based on that past experience decide how we might perform in the current situation and what the consequences of that behavior or performance might be.

Working memory provides us with an ability to profit from past experience. Regarding teenage behavior, you can probably see where we're going. How often have you asked your teen "What were you thinking?" and drawn a blank stare? Maybe the teen made a decision that you know led nowhere good in the past, and you simply can't believe he hasn't learned from past mistakes. Or even in the simpler shopping example, the teen takes all three items up to the cashier and only then finds out she doesn't have enough cash to cover the purchase. At the very least she's frustrated and embarrassed to have to figure out which item to put back. At the worst, weak response inhibition (see Chapter 9) may drive her to put the purchase on a credit card that's supposed to be reserved for emergencies, write a check her account balance can't cover, or borrow money from the friend in line with her. With good working memory, teens can juggle information in their head; people might say that they can "think on their feet." With poor working memory, teens might be described as "spacey" or "absent-minded" (they can't answer the teacher's question when called on even though they have learned the material) or as people who "don't learn from their mistakes."

How Working Memory Develops

We see the earliest examples of working memory in infancy, at about 6 or 7 months of age. When we hide an object under a blanket and the baby lifts up the blanket to find the object, she is demonstrating the earliest example of visual working memory. She can hold an image of a toy in mind and track it even though it is no longer visible. Once toddlers begin to develop language, we see evidence of verbal working memory. As a parent, one of the most striking examples of this development occurs when you hear your child give herself directions to manage her behavior. We notice that her words and even tone of voice sound suspiciously like our own. In fact, she is recalling a past situation when we gave the direction. Now, in the same situation, she recalls the direction and even the specific words and says them as a way of regulating her behavior. We can see how much more sophisticated this skill becomes by the time children reach the age of 16 or 17. A mother might say to her son, "After you finish that level on your video game, can you vacuum my car out? It's a mess from that camping trip you and your friends took this past weekend. If you finish soon enough, I can go grocery shopping now and then you can use it to go to the movies later." Recalling and following through on that demands a relatively simple aspect of working memory. We can see the more sophisticated aspect 2 weeks later, when the son remembers back to the earlier situation and says to himself, "When I took care of Mom's car when she asked me to, she was receptive to letting me use it more often. If I make sure I clean it up after I use it, she'll probably give me more leeway in how frequently I can take it." This is a more complex example of working memory in that the son goes back to a past experience, recalls his behavior as well as the behavior of others, and on that basis regulates what he will do and makes a prediction about how other people might respond.

By adolescence, teens are routinely using at least some past experiences to make judgments about what they will do in a current situation. Teens who have poor working memory are, however, those who regularly inspire the question

"What were you thinking?" and our frustration with them can lead to a lot of conflict. So working memory is important to build for a variety of positive reasons. Assess your teen's working memory using the questionnaire on page 162. Feel free to photocopy it if you want to use the form more than once, such as for another teen.

Increasing Working Memory

• *Make eye contact with your teen before telling her something you want her to remember.* While this does not guarantee that she will remember or follow the direction, it is a reasonable way to assume that at least you have her attention.

• *Avoid competing distractions when giving your teen directions.* As we noted in Chapter 6, contact with teens is fleeting, and they are frequently engaged in some preferred activity (for example, texting, Facebook, phone, TV). Parents can make the mistake of trying to give a direction while teens are engaged in one of these activities, which virtually guarantees that it will not be held in working memory. As with eye contact, if your direction is going to be effective, you need to have your teen's undivided attention, even if just for a moment.

• *If you are not sure that the teen heard you, have him paraphrase.* Use this sparingly, because it is an annoyance to most teens, even if they can do it, and sooner or later will result in some pushback.

• *Consider the timing of your directions.* The best time to give directions is not when your teen is just arriving back home from school or a night out, on her way out the door, about to go to sleep, or just waking up. The only exceptions to this rule are quick reminders about behavioral expectations with friends, curfews, brushing teeth before bed, or other things that are part of the activity the teen is about to engage in.

• *Use written reminders.* Lists, calendars, and Post-it notes, used judiciously, can be effective. They have the added advantage of defusing some of the negative emotion that might come with the verbal irritation or confrontation when parents are frustrated about tasks not getting done.

• *Encourage your teen to use or adapt technological solutions to aid working memory (for example, in smartphones, widgets, apps, or a digital calendar), or, if you are willing, offer to use his preferred technology (texting) to remind him of specific events.*

How Well Does Your Teen Use Working Memory?

For each item in the chart, first decide whether the statement to the left or right of *BUT* describes your teen better. Then rate the degree to which that statement applies to your teen. The number of items for which you chose the right-hand statement is an indicator of how much improvement your teen may need in the skill overall. Your ratings indicate possible targets for skill building: Where you chose "pretty much" or "very much" for a left-hand statement, your teen is demonstrating good use of the skill in that particular domain. "Pretty much" or "very much" for right-hand statements indicates areas that may need the most work.

Just a little	Pretty much	Very much				Just a little	Pretty much	Very much
			Some kids keep track of their belongings, like coats, keys, or sports equipment.	BUT	Other kids forget where they've left stuff and misplace things a lot.			
			Some kids are really good at remembering what they have to do.	BUT	Other kids say, "I'll do it later" but then forget about it.			
			Some kids have good ways to remember important things (e.g., lists, reminder notes).	BUT	Other kids tell themselves, "I'm sure I'll remember," but then they don't.			
			Some kids can focus on *right now* but still remember other things they need to do.	BUT	Other kids get wrapped up in what they are doing and forget other obligations.			
			Some kids know exactly what they need and make sure they bring it home from school.	BUT	Other kids forget what they have for homework or forget to bring home the stuff they need to do it.			
			Some kids seem to learn from past experience.	BUT	Others seem to keep making the same mistakes in spite of past consequences.			

• *When your teen is going to be involved in an activity or situation she has managed well in the past, reinforce that prior success as a way of reminding her to let past experience guide current behavior.* For example, "You did a good job going someplace else when some of the kids started to drink at the party you were at." You can also use negative outcomes she has experienced, but you need to do this in a nonjudgmental way. For example, "Sara, it's a Saturday night, so there will be a lot of police out on the road. We'd like to see you be able to hold on to your license and not have to pay any additional money for your insurance." If you can frame the statements in a way that reinforces past behavior or conveys that you are interested in what is best for the teen, you are reminding her of past experiences, which at least makes it more likely that she will keep that information in working memory.

Interrupting the Cycle of Forgetfulness

Stephanie sipped her coffee and listened to the news while she drove to work. She had left the house 20 minutes early after seeing her children off to school. Nick would drop his little sister, Allison, off at the elementary school before making his way to the regional high school. They ate breakfast together and talked about their plans for the day. Allison was going to a friend's house straight from school, and Nick had a dentist appointment. Stephanie had both on a planner in her smartphone, and she reminded the kids, who both sighed and rolled their eyes. Stephanie likes to be organized. In fact, her job as an office manager requires it. She almost unconsciously keeps detailed schedules and calendars for both her and her children.

Stephanie spent the day working at filing, talking to suppliers, and mediating various minor crises. In the afternoon, she called Allison's friend's father to ask what time she would need to be picked up. She was gathering her things from the office and preparing to leave when her phone rang. It was the dentist's office, calling to say that Nick never showed up for his appointment. Stephanie was irate. *I reminded him; I told him a dozen times. I do this every time. Every appointment, every conference, every hockey practice. I swear, if it wasn't for me, he wouldn't even get out of bed in the morning. Does he even think about these things? Isn't he concerned about his future? What happens when (if) he leaves the house? Who will take care of these things, take care of him? It won't be me; I won't let it. What will happen?*

Stephanie comes through the front door, having built up a good head of steam on the ride home. She goes into the living room and finds Nick on the couch watching TV.

"Nick."

"Hey, Mom."

"Hey, Mom? Umm."

"Hello, Mother?"

"What did you do after school today?"

"Got pizza downtown with Amy and then came home. Why?"

"Well, you screwed it all up."

"I what? Sorry, Mom, I don't know what you're talking about."

"I know you don't. I know that because I got a call from the dentist this afternoon asking where you were and telling me the next open appointment isn't for 2 weeks."

Nick sits up on the couch and rubs his face in his hands. Stephanie stomps through the dining room, puts her books down, and turns back to her son.

"You need to get it together."

"I know."

"You say that, but nothing gets better. You aren't on time; you can't remember anything. How can your sister or I depend on you when you act so flaky? I work. I take care of this family. I do our taxes, pay the bills, do laundry, clean the house, and cook food. I do it all, every day, on time, and yet you forget one thing you need to do."

"So what are you saying, Mom? Yeah, you made a list of everything *you* do, but how does that help me? All the time you're on me about things I need to do. 'Nick, pick up your sister. Nick, go get the milk at the store. Nick, where have all our bowls and spoons gone?' All the time, I'm expected to just remember these things you tell me, but I never get a chance to do it myself. I feel like a servant, like everything I do is just to make sure that your plan for this family goes according to your expectations."

> It is quite often the case that parents don't take into account all of the pressures acting on their child. It is important for parents to truly try to understand and feel what their kids are feeling without being invasive. Parents should try to remember what it was like for them as kids.
>
> —Ben, age 17

"Because what I want is the best for you and Allison. Without me around to keep you on track, you'd fail, Nick. I'm sure that's hard to hear—it's hard enough to say—but that's where I'm coming from. How could I believe otherwise when you fail to remember even the simplest and most repetitive tasks?"

Nick looks at her briefly while she says this, then scowls and leaves the room. She has said her piece, but Stephanie is still unsatisfied with how things turned out. She thinks for a long time about whether what her son has said has any credence. Maybe she is too on top of things. Maybe Nick is failing to remember things because

> *Nick's mom is in control of Nick's life. And if I were Nick, the second she says "Without me, you'd fail," I'd walk out.*
> —Teo, age 15

she micromanages his day for him, absolving him of the planning and the reinforcement involved in being solely responsible. Nick is bitter, and for the rest of the week the two engage in the minimum amount of conversation required.

> *If I was Nick, I would want to feel in control of my life.*
> —Lorie, age 16

A week later, Nick comes home to find Stephanie sitting at the table, watching for him to come into the room. He approaches warily and sits down. Stephanie smiles.

"I know we ran into some problems last week. I want you to know that I realize that part of wanting you to succeed is letting you take more control over your life."

Stephanie reaches into her purse, takes out a brand-new smartphone, and sets it on the table. "This is a big part of me being organized. I don't think it will solve all of your problems; I still think you need my help. But it gives you the opportunity, which is what I think you and I both want."

> *Obviously the teen is going to put games on the phone, and this may end up being a distraction, too, but I think it is better for the teen to learn how to manage distractions with responsibilities, as well as learning how to be trustworthy with tools.*
> —Tasha, age 17

> *The leap on the parent's part is a good way to establish a better relationship. Often things are messed up because neither party wants to reward the other's bad behavior, but the leap of faith gives both sides motivation to try harder for each other.*
> —Tasha, age 17

Nick smiles, hugs his mother, and takes the phone. "I promise to try harder. I appreciate you taking this leap, and I know that I will still need your help."

Stephanie shows Nick her phone, teaching him some tricks she uses when scheduling and setting reminder notices. He goes

> *The things Nick's mom gave him should let him be in control. Nick's mother should still remind Nick but slowly stop reminding him so that way he can remember on his own.*
> —Lorie, age 16

> *It is important for people to be the active drive in their own life because otherwise life loses meaning. When people aren't held responsible for their own well-being, eventually their guardian has something better to do. It is better to let kids fall while they still have a safety net to fall into.*
>
> *—Tasha, age 17*

upstairs, turning his phone on and noticing an entry for the following Wednesday, reading DENTIST. 3:30 PM. LOVE, MOM.

Q&A

Our child already has a smartphone. The problem is, she doesn't use it for this purpose. We feel stuck between a rock and a hard place. If we help her remember, she blames us for not allowing her to be independent. But if we don't help, we are afraid she will dig too deep a hole to get out of while learning working memory "on the job." How do we strike a balance between providing support and leaving enough room for our teen to develop self-reliance when it comes to her memory?

We think the most important step in getting your child to adopt these practices is to reinforce the idea that it is in her best interest to do so and that what you are invested in is the best for her. When children are young, they may mistake your encouragement for a method of control—an attempt by you to get them to do what you want. Although it is probably very clear to you that this isn't the case, your teen may see your enthusiasm as pressure to conform to a way of doing things that you endorse. This is a stretch, but drawing negative conclusions from parents' statements is something teens are very good at. So in trying to advertise a way for your teen to improve her working memory, try to present it as a positive step toward maturation. Instead of saying, "You need this smartphone," or "We think a calendar would help you remember," try "We think it is time you took more control of your own schedule. We think you're old enough to do these things by yourself." *Empower; don't admonish.* If your teen already has a smartphone, offer to sync your schedule with his calendar. This is a token acknowledgment to your teen that now he has knowledge of your daily activities, the same way you have knowledge of his.

We can appreciate the problems that Nick and Stephanie are having at home, but our teen's problems with working memory tend to make their appearance in the classroom. Specifically, our teen has difficulty remembering questions the teacher asks aloud; if she is called on, she frequently cannot recall what she is being asked, even if the question came only moments before. What suggestions do you have?

This is a perfect example of an issue that might be difficult to understand for people who do not deal with significant shortcomings in working memory. But the analogy of reading a paragraph or driving a stretch of road and being unable to remember it immediately after is something that applies in this case. The difference is that when combined with the stress of being put on the spot and the distractions of the classroom, this might happen much more frequently than with persons who have more robust attentiveness and working memory. One answer is to get your teen in the habit of writing things down. This doesn't mean that she must copy down every question verbatim. Instead, encourage her to use keywords that are important to the question and will jog her train of thought. Teens today are extremely familiar with the use of keywords due to having grown up on search engines, which are most efficient when being provided not with complete sentences but with keywords that narrow down the focus of the search. In this way, your teen is using herself as a search engine. She copies keywords in the teacher's question, then reads them back in order to trigger a search through her mind for answers relevant to those keywords.

Another practice we strongly recommend is to obtain whatever visual guides or references the teacher can offer. Whether it is outlines of lectures, highlighted portions of text, or paper copies of overhead handouts, having the subject matter of the class right there on the desk is a big help, especially if you combine these with the keyword-jotting technique. If you feel the need to go a step further, have your teen ask the teacher to write down a few of the questions or types of questions that he or she plans to ask in class. Make the teacher aware of issues relating to working memory so that he or she knows that your teen is not necessarily unprepared but just has difficulty juggling several items in her working memory.

11

....

Increasing Emotional Control

Emotional control is the ability to manage emotions in order to help ourselves regulate and guide our behavior, perform tasks, and reach our goals. When we possess this skill we can deal with life's challenges as well as its pleasures and keep cool in emotionally intense situations, from family conflicts to confrontations with a testy boss or an aggressive driver. Besides managing our temper, emotional control helps us avoid being overwhelmed by unpleasant feelings, such as irritation, dejection, and nervousness. The flip side of managing unpleasant emotions is being able to generate positive feelings as a way to overcome obstacles and keep going through difficult times. Obviously this is an important skill for our teens if they are going to negotiate the trials and tribulations of adolescence and learn to interact with a variety of different people. Having a quick temper can harm friendships and get teens in trouble at school. Being unable to pull out of a funk can make it hard to meet the demands of a tough academic schedule or perform well at sports or music. Without the ability to stimulate positive emotions in themselves, teens can find the roller coaster of adolescent life taxing.

How Emotional Control Develops

As parents, we see infants express their emotions when they coo and laugh at things that are pleasurable and when they cry and fuss when uncomfortable or distressed. When there is a good fit between a baby's needs and her parents' ability to satisfy those needs and comfort her in a consistent and predictable fashion, the baby often calms quickly. At first babies need their parents to help soothe them, but we see babies learning the skill of emotional control when they begin to soothe themselves. Some babies seem to have difficulty developing the ability to soothe themselves or control emotion in general—they continue to cry or whimper for a while after being fed when hungry, for example—and so a baby with what may become weak emotional control will often be considered "colicky" or "fussy."

As infants become toddlers and preschoolers, emotional control can be seen in how they get through the "terrible twos," with some children rarely having tantrums, others exploding regularly, and many falling somewhere in between. Children also begin to develop expectations about routines (for bedtime, bathtime, etc.), and emotional control is involved in how well they adapt to changes in those routines. So is flexibility. In fact there is considerable overlap between inflexibility (see Chapter 12) and weak emotional control. While not all children with emotional control problems are inflexible, children who are inflexible almost invariably have emotional control problems.

In elementary school, children with weaknesses in emotional control can struggle more with the increased social, academic, and behavioral performance demands and may not be able to live up to expectations that they compromise in conflicts, accept both winning and losing with grace, and understand that they will differ from some of their peers in terms of ability. If your child's lack of emotional control was recognized when she was younger and environmental modifications were made to help her, she may have been able to contain emotional distress at school, but she may still have shown a lot of emotional intensity at home.

Adolescence, of course, brings new emotional challenges for parents and teens. As a group, teens are more susceptible to heightened emotional intensity and emotional breakdowns in the face of what they consider stressful. There are both biological and developmental reasons for this. From a biological perspective, as a result of changes in the adolescent brain, teens experience a significant increase in emotional intensity. At the same time, frontal lobe development lags behind changes in other brain areas so that they have difficulty modulating or "damping down" the intense emotions they experience. Teens who have a history of weak emotional control are vulnerable to even more emotional turmoil than their peers. And if your teen is among them, you can probably expect more heated confrontations when you have differences of opinion or try to correct your teen's behavior. Use the questionnaire on page 170 to take a closer look at your teen's emotional regulation skills. Feel free to photocopy it if you want to use the form more than once, such as for another teen.

How Well Does Your Teen Regulate Emotions?

For each item in the chart, first decide whether the statement to the left or right of *BUT* describes your teen better. Then rate the degree to which that statement applies to your teen. The number of items for which you chose the right-hand statement is an indicator of how much improvement your teen may need in the skill overall. Your ratings indicate possible targets for skill building: Where you chose "pretty much" or "very much" for a left-hand statement, your teen is demonstrating good use of the skill in that particular domain. "Pretty much" or "very much" for right-hand statements indicates areas that may need the most work.

Just a little	Pretty much	Very much				Just a little	Pretty much	Very much
			Some kids stay positive even when homework is difficult or time-consuming.	BUT	Other kids get annoyed when homework is hard or confusing or takes a long time to finish.			
			Some kids can stay cool no matter what the irritation.	BUT	Other kids have a short fuse and get easily frustrated by even little things.			
			Some kids take unexpected events in stride.	BUT	Other kids get stressed out if something does not go right.			
			Some kids just let things "roll off their backs."	BUT	Other kids get hurt or aggravated easily if someone criticizes them.			
			Some kids control their temper easily.	BUT	Other kids scream or "lose it" when they get angry.			

From *Smart but Scattered Teens*. Copyright 2013 by The Guilford Press.

Increasing Emotional Control in Everyday Situations

• *Be clear and specific about your rules and keep the "have-tos" to a relatively small number.* In Chapter 6, we suggested rules in the following categories: (1) the information category: where they are, whom they are with, and whose parents are in charge; (2) the permission category: time that they need to be home and acceptable use of electronics/social media; (3) the prohibition category: people, places, and activities that are off limits. Be clear about which rules, if any, are in any way negotiable, review them on a regular basis so it is clear that your expectations have not changed, and enforce them so your teen knows you mean them.

• *Be sure your teen knows about appointments, family gatherings, and other events not scheduled by the teen for fun, so there are no surprises.* Hell hath no fury like the teen who claims not to have known about a previously scheduled, important event that now conflicts with plans he's made on his own. Because self-determination is so important to them, teens often make plans without telling parents, so putting your agenda on the table well in advance and issuing reminders increases the likelihood that teens will take it into consideration and not explode when the time arrives and they've made more appealing plans.

• *Use communication strategies that invite discussion rather than confrontation.* Go back to the communication strategies listed in Chapter 6, specifically the table that lists *dos* and *don'ts* of communication. In addition, we would again emphasize the following strategies:

> As a kid, I know that plans frequently overlap in many situations with many people. I would argue that it is all right to make plans and that occasionally it is important for parents to "roll around" my plans.
> —Ben, age 17

1. Use active listening. Active listening involves paying attention to what your teen is saying, using gestures to indicate that you understand, and from time to time demonstrating that you understand by briefly paraphrasing the gist of what the teen is saying. Listening is key. Try to avoid the urge to immediately offer an opinion, judgment, or solution to what you see as a problem. When the situation calls for it, honestly express how you feel, whether it is positive or negative, without being hurtful or insulting.

2. Negotiate whenever you can; save the nonnegotiables for situations that are important. At a time when there is no pending issue or conflict and

you both are calm and have time to talk, let your teen know that issues will come up and you will do your best to hear and respect her point of view and negotiate or compromise whenever possible. There are also times when, as a parent, you will not be able to compromise or negotiate.

3. Avoid the knee-jerk "no" to any request that your teen makes. "No" needs to remain in your vocabulary, but use it judiciously and be prepared to present your reasons.

If you can consistently use these types of communication strategies, you will at least decrease the likelihood that your teen will have an explosive emotional reaction when there is a disagreement.

Resolving Family Conflicts

Kathy hears the door slam and the lock click, and for the first time in 10 minutes she takes a full breath without speaking and leans on the kitchen counter with both hands. Her whole body is shaking, and it is not hard to see why: She and her son, Brad, have just gotten through their second shouting match of the day. Both were on the same subject, which frustrated Kathy even more because there was still no resolution, making a third battle almost inevitable. After both of them had shouted themselves hoarse and run out of steam, Brad stomped upstairs to his room to brood. It was a shame, Kathy thought, that there could not be any foresight on either of their parts that this was going to happen; they could simply have agreed to leave each other alone for the time being, but it seemed like every time Brad provoked a fight, Kathy inevitably felt she had to respond, and usually not with the answer that Brad was looking for. This time he had been invited to see a professional hockey game with a friend on Saturday in a city 2 hours away. This morning, Kathy had barely gotten the words out that they were scheduled to attend a family reunion on the same day when Brad exploded. He complained that he frequently attended family events and that the game would be a lot more fun. Kathy chafed at this and retorted that Brad was selfish and disregarded his family responsibilities. He told her that their relatives were boring, and she said that hockey was a stupid sport. She regretted this, but it felt like every time they argued, her emotions welled up and she could not help fighting back at her son, who she felt was always either being selfish or fighting with her just for the sake of it. This period of contentiousness began when Brad was about to enter high school, and now, after 3 years of it,

Kathy was worn to the point that each bout left her physically and mentally drained. It strained their relationship to the point that even when they were not fighting, she and Brad interacted under an umbrella of apprehension that the next fight was only a misplaced word away.

Kathy heard her husband, Mark, come through the door, and she felt both relief and anxiety at the sound of it closing. Now some of the anger from her son would be diverted, but it also meant that Brad would find fresh lung power to use on his father, who until now had had no part in the hockey game discussion. As Mark set down his computer and kissed her on the cheek, Kathy heard a lock turn and a door open.

"Brad and I were . . . talking earlier."

"Oh, yeah?" Mark's eyebrows went up. "About what?"

"Well, he had made plans with a friend this weekend, we have the reunion, and I told him that he is probably going to want to talk to—."

"Dad! Mom won't let me go to the game this weekend with Jessie. His dad got six seats, and Mom's complaining about some dumb thing that doesn't even matter."

"Stop right there, Brad," Mark said, "because there is something wrong with every part of what you just said."

"Oh, Jesus, Dad, not you too."

"Me too?" Mark's voice jumped up the decibel meter. "Of course me too. We've been talking about going to this reunion for months, and you agreed to it a while ago because you missed the one we went to in the summer so you could go mountain biking. I don't care if Jessie's seats are on the home bench. There's no way in hell you're going."

"Months? You guys act like you've been holding town hall meetings about this reunion every night since August. Maybe, MAYBE, you mentioned it once. Otherwise I didn't hear crap. This whole thing is BS, and I would rather stick red-hot serving forks in my eyes than go to this idiotic reunion. You guys suck. Have fun trying to kick down my door and pry my cold dead hands from my bedposts on Friday, 'cause that's what it's going to take for me to go."

Brad turned and stomped up the stairs.

"That can be arranged!" Kathy yelled after him.

> If I was Brad, I would be mad that my parents were yelling at me. When parents yell, it does not help the kid calm down and think.
> —Lorie, age 16

They heard Brad pause. Then there was a huge WHUMP, followed by a cracking sound. "Too late. I did it for you!" he yelled back.

Mark looked at Kathy. "He did not just do that."

"He did." And that weekend Kathy and Mark attended the reunion without their son. In return, they called Jessie's parents and told them that he was in no way allowed to go to the game. They took away Brad's cell phone and told him they would call the house phone every hour on the hour, and if he did not pick up, they would call the police.

> *If I were Brad's parents, I would have said he had to go to the reunion because he had an obligation, and allowing him to stay home shows that he will get his way by having a temper tantrum.*
> —Ben, age 17

> *This kid is out of control, beyond logical thinking. However, I can understand where he is coming from: Just because you say something in passing does not mean that the teen is listening. However, if he is so excited about the game, he should have made sure his parents were on board with the idea before the week before.*
> —Tasha, age 17

It took three separate attempts over the next 2 weeks, but finally the three of them were able to sit down and talk for over an hour without anyone yelling. All of them agreed that frequently the tempers they displayed did not match what was appropriate for the situation. What Mark and Kathy told Brad was that they would try to make their reactions to what he was saying as fact based as possible and that a lot of emotional interference only served to hurt feelings and degrade the situation. Brad also said that he would try to remember that his were not the only plans being made in the house and that even if his parents mentioned something in an offhand way, they meant for him to take note of it. Moreover, they agreed that Brad would be proactive in checking with them before he finalized plans with friends. They made an agreement that they would establish a family calendar and that Mark and Kathy would be responsible for tell-ing him

> *Planning is a big thing that needs to be done. Brad's parents should come up with a plan in case Brad does yell at them again.*
> —Lorie, age 16

> *I think the consequences and compromises for Brad were insufficient. They discussed how to talk about it in the future, but the scenario didn't have a punishment connected with it.*
> Tasha, age 17

what events or activities they expected him to attend. They also negotiated an agreement that before Brad finalized plans with friends to participate in some activity that was outside the bounds of his typical activities, he would check with his parents.

Q&A

We are in a very similar situation with our teen. It seems like she starts fights with us routinely and without cause. We have had moments of reconciliation, but it doesn't last, and sooner or later one of us explodes, and we find ourselves in the trenches again. What can we do?

This episode is a microcosm of parent–child relations. Everyday conflicts and disagreements all become symbols of a struggle over who is making decisions for whom. When your child was young, it was clear to both parties who was calling the shots. Children generally accept their parents' role as boss and even derive comfort from the security inherent in knowing that someone older and wiser is making decisions in their best interests. However, as we have noted, when children grow older, there is a shift in this. The lines between child and parental control are not clear; they vary with age, maturity, and context. These tensions can surface and add emotional intensity to discussions that could be nonconfrontational. We get into fights that aren't really about the issue at hand. Instead, they are driven by an ulterior conflict over control. It is unfortunate that the source of many parent–child fights is a mutual goal: both you and your teen want to see the teen accept responsibility and become successfully independent. But there is frequently a disconnect between parents and children. Parents want to keep their children from making bad decisions, while children believe that by doing this their parents are restricting their development or even insulting their sense of personal responsibility. Brad clearly wants to go to the hockey game, and his presence at the reunion is important to both his parents. This disagreement becomes a fight when it deteriorates into personal insults and rash behavior. In this circumstance, there are two issues: both sides letting their emotions get out of control and a failure to communicate. These factors are not coincidental. They have probably arisen through a long series of similar events. If you and your child allow your emotions to override what might be a relatively benign topic of conversation, both of you will come to expect the same thing in the future. In subsequent discussions, you will enter the exchange already hostile or defensive, anticipating that any negotiation will sour, and this fear creates a self-fulfilling prophecy of sorts.

The best way to deal with this issue is to acknowledge it. Try to steer the dialogue in discussions so that the focus is on the real issue and keep a constant barometer of your emotional state in mind. Remember what we said in Chapter 1 about "hot" versus "cool" cognition and the importance of parents maintaining their cool. It is especially important if your teen has a weakness in emotional control. If the conversation begins to stray or heat up, ask yourself if there is a valid reason for it or if an unrelated issue is propelling the argument. If you sense that things are going downhill, end the discussion with a promise to continue it at any other point in time. Sometimes the best course of action is to say to your teen, "Listen, I think we are both getting off track and angry over something we shouldn't be. Can we talk about this later?" Notice that this type of approach also includes you as an antagonist. It is important that you don't single out your child ("I think you're too angry to talk about this reasonably. We should do it later"). That statement implies that you are right and your teen is wrong. The first statement is also superior because it is framed as a question. Whether or not you intend to continue the discussion based on your teen's response, offering the decision to him is a subtle but effective olive branch, an acknowledgment that you respect his ability to assess his own emotional state and make a good decision.

Is there a way that we might prevent the problem from happening in the first place?

Communication is the other problem that needs to be addressed in this scenario. Teens and parents often clash over overlapping sets of plans, which may or may not have been discussed before they were finalized. One of the best ways to combat this is to have a family calendar in a highly visible place and train yourselves and your teen to use it. If everyone in the house becomes accustomed to consulting the calendar before they make major plans, this will help to avoid conflicting agendas, like the ones that Brad and his parents encountered.

Preventing these conflicts is the best possible outcome, but inevitably there will be confrontations between me and my teen. Clearly breaking your own door doesn't solve any problems. What consequences are appropriate?

It may seem extreme, but in the situation above, we would remove the door and tell Brad that he must either pay for or work off the cost of a new door. Tempers flare between parent and child, but physical violence is never a tolerable outcome. Brad has shown extraordinary rashness and disrespected both his parents' home and his own private space. So the new door will be installed when the debt is paid; until then the room remains doorless. When possible, a rational consequence that connects to the transgression is best. If it's property damage, the teen should be financially responsible. If your teen misses curfew, he must be home that same amount of time earlier the next time. Not everything has to relate directly to the incident, but it helps and reflects the real world, where often it isn't a parent but a difficult and pertinent circumstance that is the punishment.

Our teen isn't combative, but when we have a problem or conflict, she retreats and becomes withdrawn and sullen. This doesn't seem constructive to us, but it's hard to talk to someone who is giving you the silent treatment. What can we do?

While some teens are confrontational by nature, others approach conflicts with parents in a more reserved way. When dealing with withdrawn or passive, sullen teens, often the best approach is to give them time and space. You might think that your teen's ignoring you is disrespectful, but there isn't really a way to force her into a productive conversation or a sincere apology. So unless the issue is time sensitive, let her have some space and time to think. Broach the topic after a day or two in a calm manner. That said, a more prolonged period of withdrawn or reclusive behavior can be a sign of a mood disorder such as depression, and it is important for parents to recognize the signs, which include lethargy, apathy or hopelessness, fatigue, changes in sleep and eating habits, anger or irritability, and difficulty paying attention or thinking clearly. Even without symptoms like these, teenagers whose behavior changes sharply, including withdrawing from friends and family or getting involved in substance use, may be depressed. If shifts in your teen's behavior and mood have lasted for a couple of weeks, don't hesitate: call the teen's doctor and make an appointment for an evaluation. This is one area where the maxim "Better safe . . . " always applies.

12

Boosting Flexibility

Flexibility is the ability to adapt and revise plans when conditions change—when obstacles and setbacks arise, when new information becomes available, and when mistakes occur. People who are flexible are able to "go with the flow" and "roll with the punches." People who can exercise flexibility don't get thrown by last-minute changes in plans; instead of being overtaken by disappointment or aggravation, they start thinking about how they can solve the problem. Teens who haven't developed this skill still struggle with unexpected change, the way the youngest children often do. If your teen is inflexible, she may react to unanticipated change with irritability and anger.

How Flexibility Develops

In infancy, when babies have a need, they have a very vocal way of letting us know, and we respond by trying to meet their needs. We establish feeding and sleeping schedules that at first accommodate their needs, but as infants grow, they show increasing adaptation to the family's needs and schedules, and we introduce them to a variety of changes—in people, in situations, in activities—and expect them to adapt flexibly. Adaptability to change becomes a routine expectation as children are introduced to new people (babysitters, teachers), situations (day care, preschool, elementary school), and schedules (staying up late for events, spending the night at their grandparents' house). Along with this, we expect them to adjust to changes in routine without major emotional or behavioral breakdowns. Some children handle these demands for flexibility better than others. Children who struggle typically take longer to adjust to new situations, but most eventually do.

If your teenager is inflexible now, you probably recognized certain behavioral characteristics early on. Your child might have insisted on sameness and routine and probably often reacted to unexpected change with protests and tantrums. He may have had little tolerance for ambiguous or open-ended situations. Once your child set an agenda for himself in his own mind, he expected it to happen according to plan. If it did not, then some behavioral or emotional explosion occurred.

With your teen, the reaction will still be anger, but the emotion can be expressed in different ways. If you don't respond to an expectation that your teen has, often the response is that you're not being fair. Open-ended situations or tasks are described as "stupid" and a "waste of time." And, consistent with her sense of independence, your teen may well refuse to make the changes or accept the situation that you propose. If you argue the point, you activate the "hot cognition" we discussed earlier, with a resulting screaming match and door slamming.

To get a closer view of your teen's current ability to be flexible, complete the questionnaire on page 180. Feel free to photocopy it if you want to use the form more than once, such as for another teen.

Increasing Flexibility throughout the Day

While the goal is increasing flexibility as a skill, environmental modifications (see Chapter 6) still continue to play a role in the case of the teen with a weakness in flexibility. These include the following.

• *Whenever possible, provide advance notice or a warning for what's coming next*, especially if it does not conform to the teen's expectation.

• *Try to maintain schedules and routines whenever possible.* However, try to build in some flexibility at the same time. For example, rather than saying that an activity (such as dinner) is going to happen at 5:00, indicate a time range, such as 4:45 to 5:15. For appointments (dentist, doctor, etc.) let the teen know in advance that even though the appointment time is fixed, the teen should be there 10–15 minutes early.

• *Give your teen a script for handling a situation, particularly one that is*

How Flexible Is Your Teen?

For each item in the chart, first decide whether the statement to the left or right of *BUT* describes your teen better. Then rate the degree to which that statement applies to your teen. The number of items for which you chose the right-hand statement is an indicator of how much improvement your teen may need in the skill overall. Your ratings indicate possible targets for skill building: Where you chose "pretty much" or "very much" for a left-hand statement, your teen is demonstrating good use of the skill in that particular domain. "Pretty much" or "very much" for right-hand statements indicates areas that may need the most work.

Just a little	Pretty much	Very much				Just a little	Pretty much	Very much
			Some kids like the challenge of open-ended homework assignments, like writing and projects.	BUT	Other kids would rather do homework that has one right answer.			
			Some kids seem to have a Plan B to fall back on if their first idea doesn't work.	BUT	Other kids have trouble thinking of more than one solution to a problem.			
			Some kids "go with the flow" and easily adjust to changes in plans.	BUT	Other kids are thrown for a loop when an unexpected change happens.			
			Some kids can naturally "think on their feet."	BUT	Other kids need to prepare in advance.			
			Some kids can "make things up as they go along."	BUT	Other kids need to plan out in their head how something will go in advance and get upset if it doesn't happen as planned.			

unfamiliar. For example, rehearsing with the teen how to set up an appoint-ment by phone or what questions to ask on a job interview will make her more comfortable.

• *In general, whenever possible, help your teen anticipate what he might encoun-ter in a situation.* The more information he has in advance, the more comfort-able he will feel negotiating new territory.

The following strategies can be used to enhance flexibility and basically piggyback on some of the environmental modifications just mentioned.

• *Walk your teen through the new or anxiety-producing situation.* For teens with a weakness in flexibility, knowing in advance what is coming helps to reduce the anxiety and lessen the likelihood of a meltdown. Along with know-ing what's coming, they'll benefit if they can talk to you about some strategies or a script they might use to get through the situation. If you do suggest a strategy or a script, you need to be reasonably sure that it will be effective in the situa-tion. If it doesn't work, in addition to being frustrated at the situation, they will direct their frustration back at you for steering them in the wrong direction.

• *For recurring situations or expectations such as sleepovers and curfew, be clear and specific about any nonnegotiable rules.* If you have an expectation or agenda that involves your teen's participation in an activity, make sure this agenda is presented in a specific and concrete way, well in advance of the situ-ation, and as the time approaches remind her of it. As we have noted, make sure you have your teen's undivided attention when you present information like this.

• *In situations where your teen wants something from you, remember that your "maybe" becomes his "yes."* If you mean "maybe," then you need to be explicit about it, and you need to give the teen a time frame within which he will have a definitive answer to his question.

• *Assume that when your teen comes to you with a question or a proposal about some activity she would like to do, in her mind she's committed to the activity hap-pening.* While this is probably true for most teens, it takes on added emphasis for the teen with a weakness in flexibility.

• *As we have said, be judicious in your use of the word "no."* Try to save "no" for the big-ticket issues that are nonnegotiable. If the "no" you are about to say really means "not right now," then pause before you give your response, and rather than saying no, either give the teen a time when the activity can happen or give him a time when you will provide a specific answer.

• *Assume that "no" will more often than not cause a meltdown, and use the key indication strategies presented in Chapter 6 to diminish the intensity of the meltdown and your own emotional reaction.*

• *Help your teen come up with a few default strategies for handling situations where inflexibility causes the most problems.* These can include simple measures like walking away from the situation to cool off for a time and then returning or asking a specific person for help. (For example, assume your teen has recurring issues with a teacher. Rather than repeated confrontations with the teacher, a guidance counselor could serve as a good neutral sounding board.)

The Parent Said "Maybe"; the Teen Heard "Yes"

"What about this one?"

"What about what one?"

"Here: 2004 Audi A6, 110,000 miles. Heated leather seats. GPS. Dad, it's only had three previous owners."

"Three is actually a lot."

"Oh, they all probably took good care of it. I mean, it's an Audi. Right?"

John put down his magazine and looked at his daughter. "I don't know, sweetheart. Sometimes when that many people have owned a car it means there's something wrong with it. If you get the Carfax report, you'll be able to find out the accident history and stuff."

"Oh. Well, can we look at it? You said when I had $4,000 we could start looking. I finally have the $4,000, and now we can start looking. Remember? You said, 'Mei, if you show me that you can save $4,000, then I will know you're serious and responsible enough to own your own car.' Remember you said that? Well look, look at my checking account—$4,072! I have more than I even need, Dad, so can we go now?"

"Mei, Mei, Mei. Calm down. I know what I said. Listen, your mother and I have a busy week coming up. She goes to late shift at the hospital starting on Tuesday, and the restaurant is transitioning to the spring menu in 8 days, so I'll be in the kitchen all week with Jonas. Besides, you have shown me one car that is 50 miles away and in questionable condition. When you take time to find a few cars that are nearby and more realistic in terms of quality, we'll talk."

"Dad, there are like a billion cars near here listed online. Here, a 2005 Honda Civic LX. Here, a 2003 Acura TL. Here, a 2004 Subaru Impreza with a sport package and front, side, and curtain airbags. Here—"

"Mei! Enough!" John rolled up the magazine and twisted it around in his hands. "I understand how excited you are, how much this means to you. That being said, you can't do this on your own, and I just told you how busy things are this week. Maybe, *maybe*, I can free up some time in the afternoon on Friday, but I can't guarantee anything."

Mei squealed and hugged her father. She went back to the computer and alternately looked up cars and scrutinized her new license.

The week flew by. Mei went to school, did her homework, and starred and circled Friday on her calendar. She arrived home from a friend's and rushed inside, startling her father.

"It's Friday! Look, I've made printouts of four cars that I really like. I have directions, too. They're all within 5 miles of each other, and all of them meet your rigorous safety standards."

John stood with his coat in his hands.

"Mei, I'm sorry, but did I miss something? I'm just on my way back to the restaurant now. Jonas and I have prep and menu tasting before the dinner rush."

Mei dropped the papers on the table and turned a stern and anxious look on her father.

"Dad? Dad, you said that we would go on Friday. 'Friday, Mei.' That's what you said."

"I said maybe, Mei. *Maybe*."

"You said Friday. I did everything you told me to. I worked hard, I kept on target, I saved, I planned, I asked your permission, and I made a plan with you. And now you're too busy? God, Dad, it's a deal. We made a deal. Friday."

"Mei, I could say the same thing to you. Every time you need something from us, you press us to do it right away. It isn't like your mother and I are sitting on our hands telling you we can't help you because our favorite TV show is on. We're working,

> I would have done the same thing. A "maybe" to a teen is always a go . . . go . . . go!!!
> —Matthew, age 18

too, and we also ask for things from other people, but we understand that when people say maybe, it doesn't mean yes. And even when they say yes, it doesn't always mean that they are going to be able to follow through right away. I'm not saying people shouldn't be held accountable for their word, but you can't fly off the handle when things don't go as planned."

"Fly off the handle?" Mei is almost screaming now. "Fly off the handle?

I'm only treating people like I am treated. Every friggin' day I take orders from people, orders for what to do today, tomorrow, 3 months from now. And I do it, but when I ask somebody to respect my request with actions, I get brushed off. It's ridiculous! It's hypocritical! It's a double standard, Dad! I ask like an adult, but you and Mom treat me like a child!"

Mei steps to the kitchen counter, takes a glass, and fills it from the fridge. She slams it down on the table, and orange juice goes all over the printouts.

> As a kid, I might argue that it is important for parents to remember things exactly as they say it. Parents may say something, and kids interpret it differently, but the kid remembers what the parent actually said in many cases. . . . Also, I might emphasize that kids who misinterpret their parents could potentially lose trust in their parents when the real meaning of the parents' words come out and the teen thinks that the parents went back on their word.
> —Ben, age 17

"Mei, listen to what I'm saying. It's not that you don't have a reason to be upset. It's that going crazy like this isn't a productive response. And you need to realize that *maybe* isn't a promise. I told you how busy this week was going to be, and it seems that what I said went in one ear and out the other. Either way, you talk about respect, but I think that your mother and I are being realistic, not deceptive. I promise we will find time as soon as we can to help you look for a car, but you have to respect other people's plans and learn to be more flexible. It's a part of being in this family, in any family."

Mei looks at the window through the full glass of juice. She goes upstairs. Two hours later, her mother comes home to find orange-stained papers hanging by clothespins from the hood above the stove in the kitchen. There is a note on the counter that reads: *Sorry. I understand better now. I'm meeting Stephanie for lunch tomorrow, and my cross-country meet goes from 11:00 to 4:00 on Sunday. Other than that, I'm free whenever you guys have time. Love, Mei.*

A few days later, Mei and her parents

> To a teen, every "maybe" is a "yes," so when she acts out like that, it's a common response, but that doesn't make it right.
> —Teo, age 15

> Realistically, most teens would probably stay mad longer.
> —Ben, age 17

> The note two hours later is not likely to happen— maybe a note a day or two later, but not that soon after she was mad.
> —Lorie, age 16

sit down at the dining table. They decide then and there to set down some general rules for how her parents will phrase things and how she will take them. They promise, if possible, not to be ambiguous and not to say "probably" or "maybe" just to satisfy her. Mei promises to try to take the first answer they give her and accept it. When a plan is confirmed, they will explicitly say yes and try to adhere to the plan. Mei in turn will try to understand that anything but this explicit "yes" is conditional and that even then unpredictable things might arise.

> *I would be frazzled because my parent did not seem to appreciate the gravity of this moment for me. Even though Mei's father did not explicitly say "Yes, this is a blood oath for the plan for Friday," he still made no effort to modify the tentative plan once he knew that it would not work, instead leaving her hanging for the remainder of the week. The father should have recognized the significance of this moment for Mei and kept a better system of communication open for planning their adventure.*
> —Tasha, age 17

Q & A

I've had conversations like this many times with my daughter, and I just figured it was business as usual for a lot of teenagers. How do I distinguish between ordinary adolescent orneriness and a real problem with the executive skill of flexibility?

At the outset, it's hard to see that Mei has any significant executive skills issues. Perhaps she is busy and a little pushy, but any teen on the cusp of purchasing her first car is likely to act this way. The problem comes to light later in the reaction she has when her agreement with her father falls through. Mei is demanding; she perceives herself as highly organized and responsible, always accomplishing what is required of her, on time. Her world is a structured one, and when something breaks the pattern of plan, action, result, she gets very agitated. She exhibits behavior symptomatic of an inflexible teen who makes absolute plans based on conditional responses. In some ways, this problem is a good thing, and it is often indicative of a person who is naturally on top of her obligations and very goal oriented, but problems arise when her plans depend on yours. She turns her father's "maybe" into a "yes" because it makes things coherent, and she wants the plan to work.

All teens can be impatient when things aren't going their way or moving as fast as they would like. What defines the difference between these teens and ones with flexibility issues is both the frequency and degree of their overreactions. A teen with serious flexibility issues will often be inflexible, regardless of her personal interest in the activity at hand. She may get unreasonably mad at things that are out of everyone's control, like inclement weather. Although she might be unflinchingly rigid, she might expect everyone else to bend to her own schedule. The other hallmark is that when faced with a changing schedule, the teen might become unreasonably angry, even if the change is small. If a teen's inflexible attitude begins to hamper the day-to-day life of the teen or parents, then it's time to take a closer look at the possibility of the teen having a systemic inflexibility problem.

It seems very simple: I tell my son yes, no, or maybe. How come he just doesn't get it?

Teens are often under pressure from adults to do things that involve the adult's depending on the teen. Conversely, much of what a teen asks a parent to do the teen cannot do for himself; he relies on you. For example, a teen's teacher assigns homework and encourages students to attend an after-school test study group. Whether or not your teen does these things is irrelevant to the plans of the teacher. The teacher feels an obligation to help her students, but her personal plans usually do not hinge on whether or not students turn in homework on time. It is not as though the teacher cannot go home if her students don't show up, but Mei cannot go any further in her car search without her father's assistance. She is at the mercy of his schedule. So we suggest that you start by trying to understand the teen's perspective.

Then you can prevent a lot of pointless conflict going forward by laying out some very concrete rules for how you and your teen will interact with regard to future promises. Pick a time to meet with your teen—preferably not as the result of a fight, as above, but during some period of détente—and use whatever method is best, but keep it simple. One possibility is to adopt an "anything but yes" strategy. This is an agreement that no matter what is said during a negotiation, only an explicit "*Yes*, I will . . . " indicates that the plan is as firm to the parent as it is to the teen. You build on this groundwork by making sure you never use a promise or a commitment as a momentary strategy to appease your teen, and the teen agrees to try to avoid pressuring you over and over after getting an initial no. The main point is that the system you use is not as important as the consistency with which you adhere to it. Whatever you decide, you need to be faithful to it in order to provide the inflexible teen with the required predictability. In turn, your teen should understand that his hard work does not go unnoticed, but neither should your efforts be ignored.

Some parents, whether because of personality type, work schedule, or other obligations, plan their days in a much more off-the-cuff manner than others. As you might imagine, the combination of a flexible parent and an inflexible teen can be especially volatile. For instance, imagine a parent whose teen has a license but no car. The teen is able to borrow the car when the parent isn't using it. The problem is that the teen has problems with flexibility, and the parent frequently varies his after-work pattern. Sometimes he goes to the gym directly after work; sometimes he comes home first and then goes later. This infuriates the teen, who can never make firm plans that require use of the car. The solution we suggest for this problem is that you need to extend an olive branch, even if it isn't substantial. Perhaps you and your teen can agree that at the beginning of each week you will pick out 2 days, plan your car usage for those days, and stick to the plan. This way you satisfy your teen's need for structure without sacrificing your overall autonomy. Aside from that we would simply emphasize what was said above: flexible parents and inflexible teens coexist best when both parties behave consistently. Flexibility and inflexibility might merely cause friction, but when the participants fail to uphold their ends of the bargain, the results can be explosive.

13

Building Sustained Attention

Sustained attention is the capacity to keep focusing on a situation or task in spite of distractions, fatigue, or boredom. For teens, this means being able to maintain attention in class, stick with homework, and complete chores. If your teen's attention is weak, you will hear teacher complaints about the teen being off task and needing directions to be repeated. At home, you'll see your teen jumping from one task to another, often failing to finish one before moving on to a second. The teen also might seem to look for distractions such as checking Facebook every few minutes or continuously texting and responding to texts. When driving, the teen might wander all over the road and seem unaware of braking distances.

How the Skill of Sustaining Attention Develops

If we think about sustained attention as the ability to focus on a task over a period of time, we can see evidence of attention even in comparatively young infants. As long as an activity or an object is of interest or is novel, from early childhood on most of us can sustain attention. In terms of executive skills, however, we think of attention as the capacity to maintain focus even when a task isn't novel or of interest to us, *in spite of distractibility, fatigue, or boredom.* Intuitively we know that this skill takes time to develop, so we keep uninteresting tasks short for the youngest kids and also offer small rewards for sticking with them. But by the time children reach the lower elementary grades, we expect them to spend up to 20 minutes per night on homework assignments, complete chores that take about 15 minutes, and sit through a meal of normal duration with the family.

If your teen has trouble sustaining attention, you may have been hearing about it from teachers for a long time, and your child's school may have been willing to provide accommodations to help. For example, the school may have made sure that he was close to the teacher and away from the windows or chatty peers. Or teachers may have provided more frequent check-ins after directions were given or during independent work. But by adolescence, we expect children to be able to spend 60 to 90 minutes on homework, tolerate family commitments without complaining (too loudly) of boredom, and complete chores of 1 to 2 hours, even if they do need some breaks. This is a big leap forward for many youngsters with weak sustained attention skills, and when combined with the ubiquitous availability of distractions like cell phones and Internet social networking, it may result in a drop in academic performance due to incomplete homework, insufficient studying, and inattention during class. Now is the time to turn that around as much as possible, since paying attention while driving a car, once your teen reaches that age, is critical.

You can take a closer look at your teen's ability to sustain attention by using the questionnaire on page 190. Feel free to photocopy it if you want to use the form more than once, such as for another teen.

Strengthening Sustained Attention in Everyday Situations

With teens, as in the other skill areas we've talked about, negotiated solutions are best. When teens recognize their weaknesses in a situation, they are more open to problem solving. If your teen can identify particular tasks (for example, chores, homework) that are tough to focus on, talk with her about whether there are ways to modify the tasks (such as breaking them into smaller parts) that would help her maintain attention and complete the task.

• *Provide supervision.* If teens are agreeable about this, checking in with them periodically to see how they are doing or to help them get away from distractions can be effective. (This is Dick talking:) During high school, when my son was supposed to be studying for tests, he would ask me to call him periodically, just as an on-task reminder.

How Well Can Your Teen Sustain Attention?

For each item in the chart, first decide whether the statement to the left or right of *BUT* describes your teen better. Then rate the degree to which that statement applies to your teen. The number of items for which you chose the right-hand statement is an indicator of how much improvement your teen may need in the skill overall. Your ratings indicate possible targets for skill building: Where you chose "pretty much" or "very much" for a left-hand statement, your teen is demonstrating good use of the skill in that particular domain. "Pretty much" or "very much" for right-hand statements indicates areas that may need the most work.

Just a little	Pretty much	Very much				Just a little	Pretty much	Very much
			Some kids have no trouble paying attention in class, even when the teacher is boring.	BUT	Other kids lose focus in class a lot and start thinking about other things.			
			Some kids stick with their homework until it is done.	BUT	Other kids run out of steam with homework that takes a long time.			
			Some kids complete chores without having to be hassled by their parents.	BUT	Other kids start chores but don't finish them unless someone is on their case.			
			Some kids can finish projects even if they take a while.	BUT	Other kids start projects and never seem to finish them.			
			Some kids stick with things even if they get interrupted.	BUT	Other kids have trouble getting back on track if something draws them off task.			

• *Again, if your teen is amenable, ask him how long he can work on a particular task before needing a break and discuss the use of some sort of timing device to depict elapsed time.*

• *Use a self-monitoring audiotape or a tool like WatchMinder.* These devices provide electric tones or vibrating signals at random intervals as a cue to pay attention.

• *Make the task interesting.* As noted in Chapter 7, giving your teen chores that play to her interests or strengths can promote sustained attention. The objective is not to eliminate all tedious tasks, but rather to enlist the teen's help in areas where she can be both helpful to you and productive.

• *Use incentive systems.* There are basically two types of incentive systems. The first and more naturally occurring involves "first–then" plans, where after completing a less preferred activity, the teen has access to a more preferred activity. In this category are things such as homework and then computer, clean room and then use the car. The other category of incentive involves some type of pay, where a teen gets something tangible (such as money or clothes) for completing a task or series of tasks.

• *Always offer praise for staying on task and for successfully completing a task.* Instead of focusing on your teen when he is off task by nagging or reminding him to get back to work, provide attention or praise when he is on task, and also when the task has been completed.

Distracted Driver

It was a good thing the sun hadn't gone down yet, or Brian never would have found the side-view mirror in the scrub brush along the side of the road. He could not be sure what had taken it off. Most of the bushes were leafy and thin, hardly the type of thing that could take off a mirror. On the other hand, there were quite a few vines; maybe they had looped around it and that's why he found the mirror intact and relatively undamaged. Brian's ego hadn't fared so well, and even though he had laughed along with his friend at the stupid mistake, it troubled him enough to make up an excuse and call it a night. "Watch out for those bushes, man. They'll jump right out in front of you," his friend chided when Brian dropped him off. He was not sure how the mirror thing had happened; it happened so fast. He had checked his phone, shot a quick text message to his girlfriend, and suddenly his friend was yelling and the car was half off the road. Luckily, there was nothing substantial in front of them, although a few minutes after being back on the road they crossed a small, old bridge that had dry-rotted wooden guardrails; the water below was dark and looked very cold.

His friend didn't know it, but this was actually not the first time something like this had happened. The dimple in the left part of the rear bumper that Brian had attributed to a parking lot hit-and-run was actually from him bumping into a truck hitch while checking his Facebook page on his phone. And there had been others—not crashes, but close calls. Brian was thankful that he had such quick reflexes; they always seemed to bail him out of these tricky spots. Tonight's incident, though, was not going to escape his parents' notice. The mirror was intact, but the mechanism that attached it to the car was shot, and he didn't have any choice but to tell them about it.

His mom and dad did not seem really upset about the mirror, which surprised Brian. They just seemed exasperated. Brian's dad closed his laptop and looked at him. "Well, now that you've told us that, I think there's something your mom wants to say."

"Oh, okay. What's up, Mom?"

"Brian, remember 2 weeks ago when you said you were involved in a hit-and-run in the parking lot of the supermarket?"

"Well, I wasn't really *involved*. I have no idea who did it."

"Okay, you said your car got hit in the parking lot."

"Yeah . . . "

"Well, I went to file the insurance claim to have it repaired, and they called me today saying that they had a video that shows you backing into someone else's car. Now they're jumping down my throat because it looks like I lied to avoid being at fault."

Brian's father continued: "The way we see it, Bri, there's only a few things that would make someone back into another car in a wide-open parking lot in broad daylight. Either you were startled by something outside of the car or paying attention to something other than driving. We think it's most likely the latter. Would you say that's accurate?"

"Well, I didn't even look at it for more than two—"

"Would you says that's accurate?"

Brian looked down at his hands, then up. "Yeah, I guess so. I do it all the time, though, and nothing usually happens. I usually can do both."

His parents smiled and shook their

> *I would be so embarrassed to admit that to my parents. Being caught on video is awful.*
> —Matthew, age 18

heads. "You think you're doing both, Brian," his mother said, "but the truth is, you aren't; you can't. What you're actually doing is going back and forth from one to the other as fast as you can, so you think you're doing both. The problem is that—like us or anyone else—you aren't very good at this. Eventually, you get distracted for too long at the wrong time, and you'll pay for it. That's what happened 2 weeks ago. Is it fair to say that's what happened tonight?"

Brian nodded. His father leaned forward. "Bri, you're extremely lucky tonight. The parking lot was an aggravation, a nuisance. This was a near miss. You get that, don't you?"

"Yeah."

"Well, your mom and I want to try to work with you to figure out some ways to keep you from texting and other distractions while you are driving. Are there any things that you think would help?"

"I could shut off my phone while I'm driving?"

"We thought about that, but honestly, we're not sure that you'll be able to follow through with it."

"What if I put my phone in the console while I drive?"

"That's more like it, but do you think you can really do that? We want to trust you, but the first accident wasn't enough to get you to stop, so how can we know you'll follow through with this?"

"I promise, I'll really try!"

Brian's mother chimed in. "How about this? Your father and I found a software application that basically makes your phone unavailable by forwarding calls and text messages while the car is running. This means in an emergency, with the car stopped, you would still be able to use your phone, but we wouldn't have to worry about this distraction while you were driving."

"I can live with that."

> Knowing how teenagers function, he won't do it; he'll do the same thing again. I think the parents should have taken bigger strides in correcting Brian's wrong. More punishment was needed.
> —Teo, age 15

> I would feel like I had gotten away with murder, and that DWD wasn't a real threat. I would feel like I had just had bad luck once versus having extremely good luck many times.
> —Tasha, age 17

His mother added, "Because of this issue with the insurance company, I want you to call them while I'm here and explain what happened, why you reported it as you did, and assure them that it will not happen again. As far as the mirror is concerned, it would be best if we make an agreement to take a

weekly amount out of your work
check until the cost of the repair
has been paid off."

> I think the parents should have been tougher on Brian, if not through actual punishment, through extensive education on the topic. If my kid did something like this, I would make him volunteer at a hospital or view/read accounts of victims, some being people who were hurt by distracted drivers instead of actual distracted drivers.
> —Tasha, age 17

Brian knew that this was
going to interfere with his plans
to buy a new snowboard, but
he also understood that, under
the circumstances, things could
have gone a lot worse.

"I got it. Thanks, guys. I feel
good about this."

Q&A

Our daughter seems distracted even when she is driving with us, but so far she hasn't had an accident. So, do we really need to do something about this, other than remind her to pay attention?

Driver distraction is likely quite common among teens. For the general driving population, it is estimated that 80 percent of all accidents are due to driver inattention, and this is likely to be higher among teens, as are accident and injury rates. So on the one hand, even if your daughter is a simply a "typical" teen, inattention puts her at risk and is worth addressing. On the other hand, if your answers on the questionnaire in this chapter indicate an attention problem, then you have likely noticed it in other situations and it will definitely impact driving.

What can we do about DWD (driving while distracted)?

Since you won't be in the car with your teen all the time, a combination of technology and education is your best bet. As in Brian's case, there are applications on the market to disable phones while driving, and one of these should be a must for distracted teens. Newer cars are coming with warning signals for lane changes, following too closely, and potential collisions. Similar technology can be installed on most cars, and while it is not inexpensive, costs are coming down. In-car monitoring systems to check seat belt use, speeding, and unsafe maneuvering can be installed easily for under $100 per year. We have mentioned crash prevention courses, and there are Web-based courses on prevention of distracted driving that at least help teens to be aware of safe behaviors. See the Resources at the back of the book for more information.

We're fairly certain that our teen was in a small accident, but she told us a story much like Brian's: the car was hit in the parking lot when I was not around. How do we get her to tell us the truth about what happened? We're not concerned about the damage as much as we are about her safety, and we want to provide her with whatever assistance she needs to become a better driver. But we are not excited about calling our child a liar without firm proof. What are some solutions you can offer?

Unless you have independent information (from police, other driver, video, etc.) or the nature of the damage gives you a clue that something else happened, you'll need to go with the account your teen provides. We would recommend that at the beginning of a teen's driving career you discuss the fact that accidents happen, that if no other driver can be identified, you or your insurance pays the bill, and that not telling the truth can have significant legal and financial consequences. If an accident has already occurred and you suspect something, you can present the same information, explain to her that it's very important that you have the facts right, and ask (in a nonaccusatory fashion) if that's what really happened. If she sticks with her story, accept it and move on.

Sustained attention is primarily a school-oriented problem for our teen. Although he has an attention problem, the school feels it isn't serious enough to merit an individualized education plan (IEP). What can we reasonably expect from a high school in terms of helping our son cope with his sustained attention problem?

There are a couple of issues here. The first is to determine whether your child's attention problem warrants diagnosis as an attention disorder. If it does, then you are likely to have a broader range of intervention options to consider, including school interventions and medication. If you believe that your child will need systematic and ongoing intervention in school to succeed, then we recommend that you advocate for an IEP through special education in the school. Since the school doesn't seem to want to provide an IEP (but may be willing to do so once you get a professional diagnosis), requesting accommodations through a 504 plan may be an option. Both routes offer an "official" acknowledgment of a problem significant enough to interfere with your teen's education.

While your child may have an attention problem, it is possible for the school to determine that it does not have a significant negative impact on your teen's school performance. In this case, if neither an IEP nor a 504 is an option, then we recommend approaching your teen's guidance counselor and perhaps individual teachers. Guidance counselors are likely to be familiar with this weakness in teens. Because of their role in advising and scheduling, they typically will be familiar with the class requirements of particular teachers and also know which teachers are willing to make accommodations. In terms of accommodations, keep this in mind: If your teen likes a teacher or a particular subject (or ideally both!), attention will be improved because the context is rewarding. If your teen is aware of and wants to address the problem, ask him to brainstorm with his counselor or teacher to figure out what might help. Dedicated teachers are in the business of helping students succeed. Your teen's discussing the issue with teachers will make them more aware and vigilant. This can lead to simple accommodations like decreasing distractions by changing seating, monitoring cell phone use, and increasing attention through closer proximity and regular questions. Regular e-mail communication from teachers to students and parents regarding progress is important and can be especially helpful if used in conjunction with an incentive system negotiated by the teen and the parent. If problems continue, we recommend looking into the possibility of a school-based coach (see Chapter 20 for a detailed discussion).

14

Teaching Task Initiation

Task initiation is the ability to begin projects or activities without procrastinating, in an efficient or timely manner. Using this skill can involve immediately beginning a task when it is assigned or deciding when a task will be done and beginning promptly at that predetermined time. We can all identify with the urge to put off tasks we like least, but because of their context dependence teens tend to opt frequently for activities that bring more immediate satisfaction, particularly those involving peers. (Imagine your teen's response to a Saturday morning call from a friend who wants to go snowboarding or to the mall when the teen had planned to start a big history project or clean out the garage as promised.) To make matters worse, teens tend to overestimate the time available to complete a nonpreferred task and underestimate the time the task will take. (Suddenly your teen is "absolutely sure" the history project or garage cleaning will take only a few hours to finish and that there will be "plenty of time" to fit that in *after* snowboarding or shopping.) Teens with task initiation weaknesses won't just indulge themselves sometimes; more often than not they will opt for the interesting or fun activity as a way both to gain some immediate pleasure and to avoid or escape the nonpreferred task. The result? In the preceding example, sloppy, scattershot research on the history project or a garage that will remain a mess "until next weekend, when I *promise* I'll have time."

How Task Initiation Develops

When our children are fairly young, such as in preschool, we introduce them to the notion of work and chores at a relatively simple level. We direct them to clean up an area, put away toys, and the like, and we introduce the notion of "grandma's law," that the thing that is less preferred (for example, vegetables) comes before the thing that is more preferred (for example, ice cream). Most preschools reinforce these efforts by having designated cleanup routines in which all the students participate. A little later we start to put morning and bedtime routines in place and cue the children to start and finish them, which introduces the idea that activities are supposed to begin and end in a particular time frame. School gives them day-in-and-day-out experience with the importance of task initiation, and this, along with chores, continues to cement the importance of the skill.

Enter adolescence and a host of new interests—social media, video games, television shows, parties, driving—that feed context-dependent behavior. These interests and the increased freedom to pursue them serve as a direct impediment to task initiation. If we expect our teens to successfully manage the demands of school and to achieve their longer-term goals, they must be able to resist the urge to opt for the immediate "fun" activity and instead initiate work on a task that is less preferred but ultimately contributes to achieving the long-term goal. Find out how well your teen starts tasks with the questionnaire on the facing page. Feel free to photocopy it if you want to use the form more than once, such as for another teen.

Teaching Task Initiation in Everyday Situations

• *Whenever possible, use a goal that your teen has set as a way to work on task initiation.* A built-in incentive like driving or earning money will make your teen more likely to initiate a task because he has a higher stake in achieving the goal. Nonetheless, there are teens who still struggle with task initiation. If the goal is further off into the future or if the number of tasks involved in achieving the goal is large, beginning will still be a problem. However, because there is a built-in incentive, teens may be more willing to work with you on the steps to accomplish a goal.

• *If a task does not lead to a desired goal or that goal is not powerful, consider offering an external incentive.* Offer parts of the incentive along the way as the teen achieves certain benchmarks.

• *If a task seems overwhelming to your teen, encourage her to work with a teacher or perhaps to meet with you and a teacher to help break the task into more*

How Well Does Your Teen Initiate Nonpreferred Tasks?

For each item in the chart, first decide whether the statement to the left or right of *BUT* describes your teen better. Then rate the degree to which that statement applies to your teen. The number of items for which you chose the right-hand statement is an indicator of how much improvement your teen may need in the skill overall. Your ratings indicate possible targets for skill building: Where you chose "pretty much" or "very much" for a left-hand statement, your teen is demonstrating good use of the skill in that particular domain. "Pretty much" or "very much" for right-hand statements indicates areas that may need the most work.

Just a little	Pretty much	Very much				Just a little	Pretty much	Very much
			Some kids get started on homework right away.	BUT	Other kids put off homework as long as possible.			
			Some kids are good at making themselves set aside fun stuff to do homework or chores.	BUT	Other kids have a hard time pulling themselves away from fun things (video games, Facebook) to do work.			
			Some kids make a point of getting a quick start on long-term assignments.	BUT	Other kids wait until the last minute to start these assignments.			
			Some kids, if they decide they want something, start making plans right away for getting it.	BUT	Other kids spend a lot of time thinking about something they want, but never actually get started on the work needed.			
			Some kids are "go to" people when anybody wants something done.	BUT	Other kids aren't likely to be asked by others to do things because they can't be relied on to follow through.			

manageable parts, with specific deadlines for each part. Teens are more likely to initiate tasks when the task doesn't appear to require large amounts of sustained effort. If your teen is open to working with you or a teacher, have her make a specific plan for when or how the task will get done. This provides more ownership and control over the process and can have a significant effect on a teen's ability to get started without excessive complaining or multiple reminders. Again, the emphasis here is on setting small steps.

• *Let your teen decide on deadlines and on cuing systems that would work best for him to trigger task initiation.*

Managing a High School Assignment

Three months ago Lakisha was assigned a 10-page paper. For a sophomore in high school, this is a tall order. Lakisha is especially worried because in the past she has had problems completing long-term assignments. Writing isn't difficult for Lakisha, and she actually has a talent for putting together papers that read well. Lakisha's problem is that she can never seem to get started on a task. When she sits down at her computer a month before the paper is due, she sits in the chair while looking at the cursor and has difficulty imagining how she will come up with enough information to fill 10 pages. Soon Lakisha is browsing the Internet, hoping that searching for research material will inspire her. Before long, the research websites have given way to Facebook and Youtube. Lakisha gets off the computer 2 hours later, well aware that she has squandered her time but at a loss for how to overcome the problem.

With 3 weeks left until the due date, Lakisha still cannot seem to get started. She thinks about going to her teacher and requesting a change in her topic. Maybe the reason she can't get started is that she is not interested in the subject matter. But Lakisha decides not to go see the teacher, because if she did she would be admitting that she still has not started her project. She considers asking her parents for help, but she does not see how they could assist, and besides, she wants them to see her as a grownup. So Lakisha sits on the problem and spends the next week thinking about how it might get solved.

Now, with 2 weeks left, Lakisha is getting pretty worried and starts to subconsciously doubt her ability to finish by the due date, but instead of confronting her problem, she pays even less attention to it, hoping that something will come along that will get her out of her predicament. The pages of her project stay blank, but once or twice she does sit down and attempt to write. She is quickly discouraged, however, loses focus, and quits.

Fast-forward to 2 days before the paper is due. Lakisha comes home from school and finally cracks. She breaks down and tells her parents about the paper—that she has not even started it, never mind finished. Having seen this problem before, they indicate that they understand and tell her that they will do what they can to help her finish. That night, her father sits at the dining room table while Lakisha sits at her laptop. This helps keep Lakisha in the chair and off the Internet, and after struggling for 2 hours, she completes the opening paragraph. Using her father as a sounding board and editorial assistant, she outlines the remainder of the paper section by section and is able to complete four pages that night. She follows the same routine the second night, and while the paper ultimately totals only eight pages, she is satisfied that she has covered the topic in a reasonably thorough manner. When she gets the paper back with a C+ a week later, she is frustrated because she feels that she has put a lot of work into the project. In her comments, Lakisha's teacher recognizes flashes of creativity in the writing, but she notes that the disorganization and grammatical errors detract from what could be a much stronger paper. She does offer to let Lakisha edit the paper with the chance of increasing her mark by as much as a full letter grade. Lakisha initially refuses, but when her teacher offers to meet with her and talk about the changes, she decides to complete the edits and raises her grade to a B+.

Lakisha and her parents are happy with the outcome, but her parents are concerned that the larger problem remains.

"Lakisha, your mother and I are happy that this turned out as well as it did, but we haven't addressed the real issue of your getting started on things like papers in a timely fashion. Not every teacher is likely to be as willing to let you reedit or resubmit papers."

Lakisha acknowledges her parents' concerns, but she is not sure how to address the problem, and they also are at a loss. Sitting with her to minimize distractions does not seem like an effective solution.

"I know what the issue is," Lakisha offers. "I have trouble getting started, but it doesn't seem like a big deal at first because I figure I have plenty of time. Then the closer it gets, the bigger the project seems, and I have trouble starting at that point because I feel overwhelmed.

Her mother offers, "When we've got a big job to do at my office, we break the task down into smaller components and set short-term deadlines for completion of these smaller pieces. Your teacher knows the issue and seems willing

> *It is hard to break things up into small chunks with things like writing that require some momentum.*
> —Tasha, age 17

Lakisha liked the idea, feeling that it would decrease some of the stress she feels when a big project is hanging over her head. She talked with her teacher about it, and they were able to work out timelines for her next project. Lakisha also found that, as part of doing this, she

> *Fixing procrastination takes time and a lot of effort. Having been that kid all my life, I can say that doing exactly what was played out is key.*
> —Matthew, age 18

to help. Maybe when she assigns a project, she would be willing to work with you on breaking it into a series of short-term objectives with specific dates, and you can set these up in your assignment book."

> *It's a relief to have a way to overcome procrastination. I would like to see this plan used for all classes Lakisha takes.*
> —Lorie, age 16

could create outlines for these shorter objectives, which gave her a starting point for getting information down on paper, a strength of hers.

Q & A

Our teen seems to display similar problems. She can't seem to find a starting point, and the larger the assignment, the more trouble she has. How can we help her? And if this situation occurs, how can we encourage her to come to us before the eleventh hour?

Often teens with executive skills weaknesses cannot focus on a portion of the project; instead they view it as one big task, and as such it intimidates them and leads them to delay starting. This is why breaking up a large assignment into smaller component pieces right at the beginning helped Lakisha. First she found the prospect of the whole paper daunting,

> *I always feel like I do better under pressure, but I really don't. Organizing in the way presented at the end of Lakisha's story is a great way to free all of the stress and do a good job.*
> —Teo, age 15

and so she put off starting. But ending up left with only 2 days to write 10 pages was even more overwhelming. Writing one page a week for 10 weeks is something a teen like Lakisha could approach with less apprehension and more confidence.

If you think your teen is struggling to start on a paper, invite her to complete an introduction and an outline with you or with her teacher. Tell her not to think about finishing the entire piece, but to focus on writing down, in general terms, the areas and arguments she hopes to address in the body of the work. If you can get her to commit ideas to paper, she at least has a rough outline and a direction laid out.

Lakisha wasn't struggling with the process of writing itself, and maybe your daughter isn't either. But some teens who struggle with task initiation may be dealing with feelings of inadequacy about writing or about their intelligence. Don't forget, your teen may have a history of episodes like the one above. These may weigh on her mind and cause a sort of paralysis when it comes to starting a major assignment. Your teen may look back and feel that due to this difficulty with task initiation, she will not be able to commit to an idea and produce a piece of work that is representative of her true talent. In this case, your teen first needs reassurance from you and from her teacher that a good effort is all that is required. The second thing she needs is concrete evidence that she has or can find the information she needs. As a parent, you may be comfortable eliciting information from your teen about a particular subject. However, if you are not, then encouraging your teen to talk with the teacher is the better avenue to pursue. Some teens will be uncomfortable about this, feeling that they cannot explain or articulate the issue. Helping them formulate what they want to say and perhaps even working out a kind of mini-script will make it easier for them to approach a teacher, particularly if they have not done this at all or often in the past. A teen who worries about no effort or piece of work being good enough needs to start with the notion that something is better than nothing and that getting something done is better than being perfect. If everyone had to do everything to perfection, nothing would get done. Don't let your teen use fear as an escape route; not everything that she produces is the final verdict on whether her work has scholarly merit. For someone with even modest ability and task initiation problems, getting words on a blank page is the most important starting point.

We want our son to start looking for his first job. But for almost 2 months now, we've been going back and forth with him over this issue. We complain, and he says he's working on it. If we push harder, he might come home with an application or two. Our teen isn't lazy; he expresses a desire to have a job. He just can't seem to "get in gear."

This is a typical scenario for the teen with a task initiation issue. Applying for a job might seem simple to us, but to a teen it might represent a much more daunting or at least complex process: looking for available jobs, thinking about which ones might appeal to him, filling out applications, returning calls, setting up and attending interviews, making follow-up calls, and so forth. Even if a teen wasn't nervous about getting his first job (which most are), the list above can make finding employment look difficult enough for a teen to avoid it. Some ideas for finding jobs and task initiation in general include:

- *When the ball is rolling, keep it going.* Starting and stopping tasks can be the enemy of task initiation. Get your teen to spend a few hours filling out multiple applications and dropping them all off in succession. Offer to go with him. The job is done faster that way, and he won't feel like the process has been dragged out for days. It might seem self-evident, but often the best solution to task initiation problems really is to get your teen over that first hurdle and then keep him going for as long as he will tolerate.

- *Limited looking.* Suggest that your teen narrow down his job preferences before he starts looking for work. We aren't suggesting that teens have the right to be picky about jobs, but narrowing the scope of their search will keep them from getting overwhelmed. Get your teen to come up with three or four ideal job types and look into them. This is also important because of the chronological relationship between task initiation and goal-directed persistence; first you need to get a job, then you need to keep it. Getting work that you find agreeable makes all the difference in the world.

- *Stay positive.* Maintaining a generally positive attitude about your teen going through the job process is helpful. We aren't saying you need to be a cheerleader, but avoiding negative job clichés and extolling the benefits of working can't hurt your teen's willingness to start looking.

15

Promoting Planning and Prioritizing

Planning/prioritization is the ability to create a roadmap or set of steps to reach a goal or complete a task, as well as the ability to focus on what is most important along the way. Whether we're preparing a meal, beginning a new project at work, building a home, or thinking about a career change as adults we use this skill on a daily basis. For teens moving through adolescence, planning and prioritizing become increasingly important skills. On a daily basis, academics, social interactions, sports, and work may all need to be juggled. The deadline for the history project due in 2 weeks falls on the Monday after homecoming, with 12 hours of work the weekend directly before. Or the teen has to consider whether he is able to get a job so he can save for a car but still have time for a social life and manage to keep his grades up. If we were to project these concerns out over the long term, the relationship of planning/prioritizing to goal-directed persistence comes into sharp relief. For some teens the goals aren't hard to identify: I want a car; I want to be a marine biologist; I want to start a business; I want to go to the college of my choice; I want my own apartment. As a parent, you hear them all the time. And you often ask (or at least think) the question "What do you need to do to get there—to accomplish your goal?"

The answer that you get can be instructive on a number of levels. If you don't hear a plan or a set of priorities or see the teen's roadmap, then planning/prioritizing is the issue. Or maybe your teen actually has a plan and maybe even a starting point. But as the days, weeks, or months pass, he doesn't get started on it. If that's the case, then task initiation may be the issue. Or your daughter does get started and is gung ho and all fired up in the beginning! But then other interests come along and the enthusiasm wanes. Here maybe sustained attention is the issue, or maybe the goal has lost its glow, and it wasn't really that strong to begin with. Or maybe she needs more benchmarks to see that she is closer to her goal. Other teens have trouble with longer-term goals. If you have a teen like this, he is likely to set context-dependent goals that have a more immediate payoff. In this case, you can work on planning and prioritizing, but it needs to be in relation to your teen's shorter-term rather than your hoped-for longer-term goals. Those will need to come later.

So planning and prioritizing are not only important skills unto themselves but also a window into the other executive skills that come into play if a goal is to be achieved.

How Planning and Prioritizing Skills Develop

When our children are young, we take on both the planning and prioritizing roles for them. We (and their teachers) decide on priorities, small and large, let our kids know what these are, and then typically help them formulate the plans to reach a goal. At young ages, at home, this involves telling them a series of steps to follow. At school, it comes in the form of externally organized schedules and routines that, depending on the classroom and the teacher, children are increasingly expected to learn and follow on their own. At home, verbal directions are gradually replaced with lists or checklists of steps for kids to follow to accomplish a task. By the upper elementary grades, we expect our children will be able to make plans to do something special with a friend or figure out how to earn or save money for an item of moderate cost. By this point, they can also carry out longer-term projects in school, as long as the steps are broken down by a teacher. By middle school, they can make plans for extracurricular activities or summer activities and can do research on the Internet for projects at school or to learn something of interest. For adolescents, the expectations for planning extend to areas like finding jobs, selecting courses to meet graduation or college requirements, and meeting deadlines for SATs and college applications.

Two factors separate planning and prioritizing in adolescents from these skills at younger ages. The first is that at least some of the significant goals of teens (particular jobs or careers, college, purchases of big-ticket items such as cars) are complex and at some distance in time from the present. This means that the planning process is also more complex and plays out over a longer period of time than what teens may be accustomed to. This problem can be exacerbated when your teen sets goals that you don't agree with and then needs your help in planning the steps to achieve them. Examples of this might include post-high-school plans, purchasing undesirable vehicles, or pursuing dangerous activities. The second factor has to do with prioritizing. Once you've been prioritizing for your child for years, it can be tough to stop doing that in mid- to late adolescence. Yet your teen probably has her own priorities at this point and will push back if you try to dominate these decisions. Many parents find that the tug of war over priorities becomes a major source of conflict. Not only might you put certain goals ahead of the ones your teen values most, but your teen may balk at having to consider your priorities (safety, finances, etc.) as part of the planning process for reaching a particular goal.

It's in planning and prioritizing that negotiation and compromise become critical to success. As we've already discussed, you may need to work with your teen's priorities as opposed to focusing exclusively on the priorities that you've set for him.

Use the questionnaire on page 208 to evaluate your teen's planning and prioritizing skills. Feel free to photocopy it if you want to use the form more than once, such as for another teen.

Promoting Planning and Prioritizing in Daily Life

• *Use the things your teen wants as a jumping-off point for teaching planning skills.* Any goal that requires a roadmap to achieve can be used to teach planning skills, but your teen is going to make a higher investment in working toward personally meaningful goals. So, obviously, saving money for a ski trip with friends might be more motivating than writing the essay that counts for 20% of his English grade. But you know that the essay has to get done, so think about how you can build in incentives centered on things your teen values. Offering time incentives is an example. If your teen has a license but no car, offer her the use of yours in exchange for progress on her essay. "Jan, if you write five pages of your English paper tonight, you can use my car all day on Saturday." You can't always make the task more pleasant, but you can create positive incentives that make the task more worthwhile.

• *Spell out in advance any priorities or limitations you want to impose on a goal that is more important to your teen than to you.* For example, if your teen wants to purchase a car and you have specific safety or financial considerations or limitations in mind, discuss them with your teen before he begins his planning

How Well Does Your Teen Use Planning/Prioritizing Skills?

For each item in the chart, first decide whether the statement to the left or right of *BUT* describes your teen better. Then rate the degree to which that statement applies to your teen. The number of items for which you chose the right-hand statement is an indicator of how much improvement your teen may need in the skill overall. Your ratings indicate possible targets for skill building: Where you chose "pretty much" or "very much" for a left-hand statement, your teen is demonstrating good use of the skill in that particular domain. "Pretty much" or "very much" for right-hand statements indicates areas that may need the most work.

Just a little	Pretty much	Very much				Just a little	Pretty much	Very much
			Some kids are great at figuring out the steps needed to do a project.	**BUT**	Other kids don't know where to start or how to make a plan.			
			Some kids know what's important or what needs to be done first.	**BUT**	Other kids have trouble prioritizing when they have a lot to do.			
			Some kids make a plan for the day either on paper or in their head.	**BUT**	Other kids let the day unfold and then realize afterward that there was stuff that didn't get done.			
			Some kids divide an assignment into pieces and stick to a timeline.	**BUT**	Other kids work on long-term projects in spurts without any real timeline.			
			Some kids are good at figuring out ways to save money for something they want.	**BUT**	Other kids want expensive things and don't know how to go about saving money for them.			

From *Smart but Scattered Teens*. Copyright 2013 by The Guilford Press.

process. Similarly, if your teen wants to attend a particular college and there are financial constraints, the teen needs to know this before the planning process begins.

• *Involve your teen as much as possible in the planning process.* Once you have established whatever priorities or limitations you want to attach to a goal, some teens can go off on their own with a minimum amount of direction from you. They may be able to consult with friends or teachers or gather information on the Internet and bring it back for discussion. If your teen can't do this, try to lead her through the process by asking questions rather than simply telling her what to do. If she can't come up with suggestions on her own, then asking questions and providing choices that she can select from will help her maintain active problem solving in the process.

• *If your teen appears to understand the various pieces of a project that need to get done but isn't sure how to get started, prompt him to prioritize by asking what needs to get done as the first step, the next step, and so on in the process.* If your teen is unsure, again offer him choices and discuss the implications of his choices with him.

Making a Purchase

"Ready?"

"Almost."

"Come on, you've been sitting at that thing all morning." Samantha grabbed her dad's arm and tried to yank it away from the laptop.

"I know, Sam. Trust me, I wouldn't be here if I didn't have to."

"What are you doing anyway?"

"Well, it's getting to the end of the month, and the end of the year is coming fast. I'm trying to start getting our finances in order. We have to think about paying for your brother's next semester at college or at least helping him find loans. We are talking about going to Florida with Ashley and her family during winter break. That won't be free, and I'm guessing you don't have a lot of money lying around. We're also thinking about switching banks and refinancing the house. It takes a ton of planning to make sure these things go smoothly."

"Don't forget Christmas presents and looking for a car for me."

"Shoot. I was hoping you would forget about those two," her father said grinning.

"Not a chance. Let's go, though. I need to get this poster board because my project is due tomorrow."

They left the house and drove down a few side streets until they got to the main road, lined with department stores, dealerships, and chain restaurants.

"Have you thought any more about the car you want and how you're going to get it?"

Samantha squirmed a little. "Not really. I mean, I'm working 15 hours a week sometimes, and I've saved about $5,000. That seems close enough. I've seen cars around for less than that."

"Mmm . . . Do you still have the list we gave you? It's your money and your car, but Mom and I did have a few requests in terms of safety, and we would prefer you don't get a bare-bones insurance policy."

"Yeah, it's around somewhere, and Mom said you guys would help me with the insurance?"

"Yep, but you have to call our insurance company and ask what your rate would be. Don't forget, that becomes part of your cost."

"Well, I figure that I have $5,000 and still have my job. If I keep the job, I can get a $5,000 car, then pay my insurance with the job. I don't know. It will all work out, I'm sure."

Samantha's dad just nodded and kept driving. They got the poster board and headed home.

A couple of hours later, Sam's dad knocked on the door of her room and went in. He walked over to her desk and looked at the collage of papers, pictures, and electronic devices spread out across her desk. He tapped her on the shoulder, and she jumped, then took off her headphones and looked up at him.

"Yeah?"

"Can we talk for a minute about this car thing?"

"Sure, Dad."

"Well, I'm concerned that maybe you haven't thought out your plans for buying and maintaining one as much as you should have. When we talked earlier, it seemed like you weren't really sure of what you wanted or needed, and I don't want to reach a point where you actually need a car and can't get one because you didn't prepare properly."

"Yeah, I hear you. I guess I just never really thought about where to start. It seemed simple. I just save up the money and buy a car."

"I know it might look like it's that easy, but in reality there are a lot of details that need to be covered. Mom and I will help you with that for sure, but we want you to understand it so it will turn out the way you want."

"Okay, well, what are you suggesting?"

"How about you do what research you can about cars you might be interested in but also meet the safety concerns we talked about? When you come up with a good list, we can sit and discuss the ins and outs of car ownership. Cars require maintenance. Drivers need insurance. You said you had $5,000 saved up. I suggest that, first and foremost, you don't focus on cars that cost $5,000. See if you can find something a little less expensive, and that will leave you some money to work with if there are still unexpected costs."

> *I think I would have been excited to do the research on cars. It's a good way to get kids to realize how expensive things are, and having Sam do the work will benefit her eventually, but I think the dad could have taken a more helpful approach and maybe sit with her and do the research.*
> *—Teo, age 15*

"Okay, Dad. Sounds good. You know, though, I could probably get more bang for my buck if I bought a motorcycle . . . "

Sam's dad feigned banging his head against the wall and then patted her on the shoulder. "Let's try mastering four wheels before two, okay?"

> *I wouldn't mind getting the list of cars if my parents helped me with the rest. Planning for the car helps us accomplish our goals in the future as well. Having Sam do most of the planning will be a good thing.*
> *—Lorie, age 16*

Q & A

As much as we wish that our teen had saved the money on his own, the truth is that we will be paying for our son's first car. Sometimes we think he really doesn't understand the costs involved; other times we feel like he is jousting with us about how much we are going to spend on him. All we know is that he doesn't seem to be showing much gratitude, and we're wondering if we should just put off the purchase until he shows signs of understanding what a big deal investing in a car is. Should we?

It might be a good idea to postpone the purchase if you think your teen has no idea how significant an asset a car is, because without that knowledge he's not likely to be as careful with the car as you undoubtedly want him to be. But to delay just because the teen should be showing more respect and gratitude will probably result only in a lot more conflict. If you think your teen doesn't fully understand not only the cost of a car but also the other expenses involved in owning a car, be proactive in investigating how much he does or doesn't know. Some teens, like Sam, can formulate a goal and even prepare to reach it, but they lack the proper orientation, information, and strategy to get all the way there.

When we're doing something we've never done before, we all need the help of others. What can be different in teens lacking executive skills is that they don't know what help they need or whom to ask for it. It's also possible that they aren't aware of their own lack of knowledge about the issue. Part of Sam might believe that this "winging it" attitude is how all people go about making important decisions (and unfortunately, some do!). But note that when Sam seemed to have a lack of knowledge and direction, her father didn't scold her for being ignorant or just tell her to figure it out; he didn't assume that she was just trying to get to him. He took the opportunity to seek out how much she knew and then educate her.

> *I would be happy that I had freedom to pick my first car within reason. Sam seems to be pretty independent; I can see where Sam would want her father to be part of the decision, however. I feel like sometimes it is nice to have someone to sit up with you and be with you when you make big decisions. Maybe this reflects on my personal dependence on my family, but I would want my family not necessarily to make the decision for me, but to be with me when I made the decision.*
> —Tasha, age 17

Sam had already saved the money, so we know she wasn't lacking in desire for the car or willingness to work hard toward her goal. But allowing her to proceed on her own could put her in over her head, ruining the experience and tarnishing the lesson that her hard work had paid off in the end. Sure, if your child hasn't saved a dime or seems indifferent to your help, she might have a problem with goal-directed persistence (see Chapter 18) or motivation. But the circumstances here tell us that this isn't the case with Sam. It's an important thing to recognize because it will help you avoid potentially offending your son by mislabeling his poor planning skills as sloth and tailor a solution geared toward introducing and reinforcing the various steps and angles that need to be considered, which he will then apply to future situations on his own.

Most parents do want their teen to pursue goals like getting a driver's license and car. But what if a teen wants to pursue something that parents don't agree with? Our teen has recently begun saving money in order to take a year off after high school to work and travel, with the intention of going to college the following fall. She's approached us looking for both approval and funding, either outright or through selling a car we purchased for her. Our biggest concern is that this break will continue past its set time frame and our teen will never go back to school. We don't really have a problem with our daughter not attending college right away, but we are afraid that she will put off going back indefinitely. Basically, we are worried that if she goes out on her own and earns some money, she will get caught up in the moment and forego returning to school in favor of protracting this post-high-school vacation. If she alights on some passion during this time that doesn't require her to have a degree, fine, but we are scared that naïveté or lack of long-term foresight will strand her in an educational and career limbo—that she is, in a sense, opening a door behind which the grass looks very green to an 18-year-old, but in 3 years it might not be so appealing, and she will turn around to find the other doors shut as well.

This is not an easy situation to navigate by any means. Your teen depends on you both financially and as providers of advice and love. But she is also on the cusp of legal adulthood. This question really has as much to do with whether your views about this situation diverge from your teen's views as it does with planning and prioritizing.

Ultimately, your teen is becoming an adult, and the final choice rests with her. This doesn't mean you have no recourse, but it means that above all you need to respect that this decision resides fully in your teen's jurisdiction.

Being aggressive and forceful isn't a good idea. In fact trying to berate or intimidate your teen might turn her off to your point of view. Creating a power struggle takes the focus away from the issue at hand and makes it an abstract, rhetorical argument about independence.

We recommend that you calmly approach your teen and lay out your reasons for objecting to the goal. Make her aware that you respect her independence. Make her aware of the opportunities that might be forfeited as a result of her decision (college acceptance, scholarships, financial aid, work study, housing preferences, etc.). Finally, you may choose to tell your daughter that it is your desire that she go to school, and while you are willing to contribute financially toward that goal, she will have to fund this venture on her own. Your goal is not to be punitive, and your tone shouldn't sound dictatorial. Your focus should simply be to acknowledge your teen's independence, as well as your own.

16

Fostering Organization

Organization is the ability to create and maintain a system for arranging or keeping track of important things. For most of us, the benefits of organizational ability are clear. Keeping track of things and having a reasonably organized home or work environment increases efficiency by eliminating the need to waste lots of time looking for things just to get ready to work on a task or project. This in turn reduces stress. Think of the last time you lost your keys. You probably went from 0 to 60 in terms of stress as you frantically searched for them. For teens, lack of organization can be particularly stressful because, as noted in Chapter 14, they tend to overestimate the amount of time they have to do tasks or meet deadlines and underestimate the amount of time tasks will take. As a result, they are usually operating pretty close to the edge to begin with, and not being able to find critical materials (keys, books, phones, etc.) can send them over the top in terms of stress. Since parents are often on the receiving end of this ("Where'd you put my backpack?"), it is important both for us and for our teens to learn some organizational strategies.

How Organizational Skills Develop

As with most of the other executive skills we have talked about, at first we give our children a lot of help with organization: We provide our children with structures that they need to keep their bedrooms and toy areas neat, such as storage bins, hampers, and bookcases. At school, their teachers provide them with cubbies, desks, spaces for outerwear, notebooks, and more. Many of these efforts benefit adults most initially, but they are also intended to help children understand how to organize personal belongings and the necessary materials and tools to get work done so that ultimately they can do it on their own. We walk them through the steps of room cleaning ("Let's start with you putting your shoes in the closet" and then "Now, let's put all your trucks in the truck box"). We also try at least to establish rules for children who are a little older, such as "no drinks in the living room" and "put your dirty clothes in the laundry basket before you go to bed." Once they reach school age, teachers and parents are working on skills such as notices and permission slips going back and forth from school and sports equipment being in specific locations. By 9 or 10, we are expecting children to keep track of homework and materials, and by middle school, we expect them not to lose sports equipment, instruments, or personal electronics.

Gradually we try to step back as parents from step-by-step and moment-to-moment monitoring and supervision, hoping to get by with occasional prompts. By late middle school or early high school, we expect our children to take over maintaining these organizational systems on their own, but in many cases teens are more conscientious about this in some areas than others. For example, a teen who doesn't want to be benched for a game will be much more likely to take the required sports gear to the gym than the same teen might be to remember to take homework to school. A teen who likes playing in band but dislikes practicing clarinet might develop a suspicious habit of "forgetting" to bring it home from school. Evaluate your teen's organizational skills using the questionnaire on page 216. Feel free to photocopy it if you want to use the form more than once, such as for another teen.

Fostering Organization in Daily Life Domains

Unlike some of the other executive skills, your teen may be more open to accepting help with organization from you because it's usually in his interest to be able to find what he needs. But teens are more likely to welcome your providing structures and strategies if it doesn't involve your directly moving or manipulating their personal belongings, particularly in what they consider to be the private space of their rooms, except maybe when setting up the original system. This means that for any organizational schemes or strategies, your teen has to be an active and willing participant, and if organization involves their personal belongings, they must first give you explicit permission to touch these belongings.

How Well Does Your Teen Use Organizational Skills?

For each item in the chart, first decide whether the statement to the left or right of *BUT* describes your teen better. Then rate the degree to which that statement applies to your teen. The number of items for which you chose the right-hand statement is an indicator of how much improvement your teen may need in the skill overall. Your ratings indicate possible targets for skill building: Where you chose "pretty much" or "very much" for a left-hand statement, your teen is demonstrating good use of the skill in that particular domain. "Pretty much" or "very much" for right-hand statements indicates areas that may need the most work.

Just a little	Pretty much	Very much			Just a little	Pretty much	Very much
			Some kids keep notebooks and backpacks organized to find things easily.	**BUT** Other kids can't find things in their notebooks or backpacks because they're a mess.			
			Some kids are naturals at keeping their bedrooms neat.	**BUT** Other kids seem to never clean their bedrooms unless someone forces them to.			
			Some kids make sure that their desks are cleared off before they start working.	**BUT** Other kids work at desks that are piled high with clutter.			
			Some kids know exactly where to find important things (cell phones, keys, etc.).	**BUT** Other kids lose or misplace important things a lot.			
			Some kids put their things in a specific place as soon as they are finished using them.	**BUT** Other kids leave their belongings all over the house (or even at other people's houses!).			

From *Smart but Scattered Teens*. Copyright 2013 by The Guilford Press.

> *Many times the biggest problems that go along with organization are getting started, knowing where to start, and having the resources needed to change.*
> —Ben, age 17

If organization is a particular strength of yours, we offer a special note of caution. What seems easy and even self-evident to you might be quite challenging for your teen. Disorganized teens are often oblivious to the mess around them, and as a result, you may need to modify your expectations.

• *Like most of the other executive skills and routines discussed in this book, with teens organization is best approached from some area that they have an investment in.* This might involve sports, school, or a job, if there are dress or uniform requirements. If your teen is struggling and you are on the receiving end of the stress ("I can't find my keys, homework, cleats, running shoes, shin guards, cell phone, etc."), offer to help. If the teen cannot come up with an idea for how to better manage the situation, give him a couple of different options and let him choose the one he likes.

• *In the short run, even though it might seem counterproductive, offer reminders in a format that your teen feels she can tolerate.* This might mean personally going through a checklist with her just before she leaves, posting a visual, sending a text, or creating a personalized application on her cell phone. Over time, this needs to fade to something that is not directly dependent on you as the agent, but with practice you and your teen will be able to do this.

• *Even though you feel it is solely your teen's responsibility, periodically offer to help him clean and organize his space.* As long as the teen is working with you and you are soliciting his ideas, assume that he will benefit from the practice.

• *Model some simple organizational schemes for your teen.* If you are constantly losing your keys or cell phone, any attempt on your part to talk with the teen about her organization puts you in the category of "talk the talk" rather than "walk the walk."

"I Can Never Find My Stuff"

Seven pairs of pants times four pockets per pair, plus two jacket pockets, is . . . 30 pockets. Jamie thought about this as he ran through his room, taking jeans off the floor one pair at a time and clapping each pocket between his hands, then throwing them into the stack on his bed. After going through all seven pairs, he spun in space, looking around the room. *There's got to be another pair somewhere.* He grabbed the baseball bat leaning against the nightstand, dropped to his stomach, and used a sweeping motion to clear everything out from under his bed. An iPod, four Q-tips, a pair of nail clippers, and three balled-up dirty socks came flying out. *Nice.* He grabbed the iPod and nail clippers. *I've been looking for those forever.* He stood back up and froze. *Wait, now what was I looking for again? Hmmm . . . not the iPod, not cleats, not nail clippers, not headphones.* He stood still as if the idea would bounce out of his head if he moved. *Not medication. Not a belt. Not sunglasses . . . KEYS! JACKET!* He flew over to the desk, ripped the jacket off his chair, and tore down the stairs. He grabbed his bags, and just as he was reaching the door, he froze again. *You're sure they're in the jacket?* He dug his hands in and found nothing but empty pockets. *Shoot, shoot, shoot. Other jacket, maybe?* Jamie went to the closet and rifled every pocket in it, even his parents'. Nothing could be found but loose change and a card from the doctor with an appointment for tomorrow that he had completely spaced on. *Phew, well that's a plus.* He went to the kitchen counter, where there was a bowl of miscellaneous items: paper clips, old matchbooks, golf ball markers, lanyards, and pennies. Not there either. Jamie scanned the counter, picking through loose mail like he was playing three-card monte. The keys peeked out from under a stack of junk envelopes. Jamie grabbed them and ran out.

He had gotten to school before he realized that his backpack was sitting on the kitchen counter. There weren't any major assignments due that day, but Jamie didn't have his homework for three classes, and he had worn his repertoire of excuses pretty thin. Some teachers even seemed to approach him wearing a look like they expected him not to have whatever was due that day. When he got home that night, his parents confronted him. This had been going on for some time, and his mom and dad had requested that Jamie's teachers e-mail them when he missed multiple assignments.

"Jamie, we understand that you were tardy today, and you didn't have your homework for Mr. Carmichael, Mrs. Trist, or Mrs. Minier. What happened?"

"Well, Mom, I couldn't find my keys this morning, and when I finally found them, I was in such a rush that I ran out without my bag. The homework is done, honest. I just left it all here."

"That's almost worse, Jamie," his father said. "You went to the trouble of doing the work, but no one will know if you cannot produce it on time. This seems like a growing problem. Your mother and I don't want to see you getting grades you don't deserve, just because you can't remember things. There have been days when you forget a belt, or spent 30 minutes looking for something that was in your pocket. Remember that day when you had to wear mismatched shoes to school in order to turn that paper in on time, because you couldn't find the other shoes? Remember when they turned up in your car?"

Jamie chuckled, then drew it back. "Yeah, I remember. It's funny now, but at the time I was so embarrassed, it was all I could do to walk into the building."

Jamie's mom cleared her throat. "What if we offered to help you out? Remind you when your assignments were due, make sure all of your stuff is in the right place?"

> *If I was Jamie, I would like some tips but not many at once, or else I would feel like a kid instead of a teenager.*
> —Lorie, age 16

"I hear you, Mom, but I'm not 6 years old anymore, either. If you guys keep doing that kind of stuff for me, I won't learn to do it on my own."

"We understand that, Jamie," his father said, "but we feel like our job right now is to get you to the end of high school with grades and teacher recommendations that reflect your true talent."

> *Being just like Jamie, I can relate. Having active parents isn't fun now, but the later outcome is so much better.*
> —Matthew, age 18

"So what about when I go to college, then? You guys won't be there to put my backpack in my hands or remind me when a study group meets."

"True," his mother said. "What about this? We start here and there, helping you with what all of us decide are the most critical things. If this helps, we will pull back. If it doesn't, we will help you with a few more things until you get the hang of it. Our goal is to not be hostile toward one another, and to give you some flexibility to become self-sufficient. We just don't want to see you dig a hole now that you can't get out of later, Jamie."

Jamie nodded. They talked more and in the end decided that in the immediate future his parents would make sure that Jamie's backpack was by

> *Having Jamie create a checklist would be a good idea.*
> —Lorie, age 16

> *I would feel dumb and childish if my parents offered to check on my backpack and keys. I think just giving him pointers was enough to help him.*
> —Teo, age 15

the door and his keys were on the key hook every night. They also gave him some ideas for things to try on his own, such as wrapping his headphones around his iPod and leaving it in one of only two or three places. That way, if he was missing it, he would know right away to look at his computer desk, the kitchen counter, or the console of his car.

Q & A

Our child is defensive about taking our reminders. He can't help feeling like we are regressing in the way we honor his independence.

This is a case of you and your teen sitting down and facing some facts. Right now, your teen simply is not capable of managing things on his own. He can't expect to exercise complete control over his life, and you aren't going to be able to fix everything at once. The case in the story above spells it out; resolving this problem is about compromise and helping your teen gradually create systems and then practicing them enough to become more independent. We recommend that you all start with the most important things. Jamie's most glaring issues are losing his keys and forgetting his school materials. If he and his parents can work to solve these two problems, this will go a long way in alleviating the run-ins with teachers and the associated stress on everyone involved.

Visual cues (for example, checklists) work better for some kids than verbal reminders. Aside from the fact that they are always present, they don't involve you directly reminding your teen. Some teens, even if they acknowledge needing the help, will feel like you are nagging if you are always telling them to get their materials organized. The downsides of visual reminders are the same as the pros, however. If visual reminders aren't followed, but they are always present, they may lose their significance or the ability to catch the eye of your teen. The bottom line here is that the disorganized, in the short run, will need practice in both creating and maintaining organizational schemes (like putting keys reliably in the same place).

> *As someone who struggles with organization, I would be grateful for help at times. However, if it became over-the-top, I would be angry at the infringement on my independence. However, when it got to a point that I was frustrated, I would verbalize my dilemma and hopefully my parent would cue in and back off. The slow weaning of dependence will help the kid figure out what he wants for himself.*
> —Tasha, age 17

We're now in the midst of helping our teen remember things that are vital for school. But long term we know she will need to be totally independent. How do we transition responsibility without things falling apart?

Okay, let's suppose you have successfully arrested the progress of the problem and allowed your teen to stabilize her life. Now it's time to think about how to gradually give back the job of remembering things to her. First, make sure that you, your teen, and anyone else involved (for example, your spouse) is aware of the goal. It is not about one day turning off the switch and playing the wait-and-see game to see if your teen has assimilated the habit. If your assistance with organization has been reasonably successful, then talk with your teen about beginning to pull back on the assistance. This means slowly fading the reminders. This might go from a verbal reminder before leaving for school in the morning to a reminder about getting things ready the night before as part of a regular routine. You can also go from verbal reminders to something more visual that does not require your immediate presence, like a Post-it on the bathroom mirror. In our high-tech world, smartphones represent a kind of technological surrogate frontal lobe. It is possible to program alarms with written and even auditory reminders about materials and events to be remembered. If you work with your teen to make a list of the critical things that she needs to have before leaving in the morning and she programs these into her phone with alarms she has chosen, she will have the reminders she needs but be able to set them up independently.

Our teen never had a serious problem with organization in terms of remembering his schoolwork or functioning as any other normal teen might. But his room is just really messy. He seems to be able to find everything, but as highly organized parents, we find his messiness aesthetically annoying and can't help feeling paranoid that his "system" will one day fail him. What should we do?

Unfortunately, the short answer is that you should let him be. Sure, we may find it annoying that teens leave things on the floor or spread papers all over their desks. But if it isn't impacting your teen's life outside of his room, then there isn't really a cogent, valid way for you to rationalize forcing him to be clean "just for the sake of it." That said, your teen's room isn't a fortress that you have no control over. We don't believe that permanent alterations made to a room (painting, etc.) can be done without your consent. And if organization or sanitation becomes a concern, you are clearly justified in intervening. But as your teen grows, part of honoring his increasing independence involves compromise on your part in respecting the privacy of his personal space.

> *A lot of kids would argue that organization is different for each person. I may not be as organized as others, but I know where my stuff is and my own personal system may work best for me.*
> —Ben, age 17

One caveat to this, however, is that it won't always be just you and your teen (and perhaps close friends) seeing that room, and your teen won't always live there. While keeping your distance is a sign of respect, also make sure your teen is aware of the fact that peers (including potential significant others and future roommates) might have a different opinion on what constitutes a habitable space. By stressing this point, and not focusing on differences between you and your teen, you are respecting the teen's space while also teaching him that in the not-so-distant future it will be in his best interest to reevaluate his cleanliness standards.

17

···

Improving Time Management

Time management is the ability to estimate how much time is available, how to spend it, and how to stay within time limits and deadlines. It also involves a sense of time urgency—that is, the notion that it is important to accomplish particular tasks within a designated time frame. If this is a strength for your teen, she is able to estimate accurately how long a task will take and how much time she has to complete the task, and then adjust the pace of her work to meet time constraints. The teen usually meets whatever deadlines have been set, such as those for homework assignments, and does not routinely overextend herself.

It's important to note, however, that this may be an overly idealistic picture even for teens who are strong in this executive skill. Nowadays, time management seems difficult for most people because the demands of school or work and personal life typically exceed the time available to complete them without chronic sleep deprivation. Nowhere does this fact of modern life seem more evident than in teenagers. They need to spend a lot of time on schoolwork, yet they don't want to miss out on social events, they might want to compete in sports or engage in other pursuits, and they often feel pressured to achieve to qualify for the college of their choice or other post-high-school plans. So even with good time management skills teens can be stretched beyond the limit of the 24-hour day, and things may fall through the cracks as a result. The trick for parents is to distinguish these kinds of inevitable problems from the more serious time management issues that indicate a lagging executive skill: teens who miscalculate how long tasks will take, have difficulty sticking to a schedule they have set, and chronically "run late."

How Time Management Develops

The development of time management begins in early childhood, with parents initially taking the lead. We prompt our children when it is time to get ready for school or bed, and we adjust our plans and expectations, taking into consideration the different speeds at which children work. Initially, children tell time not by the clock but by sequences of events that occur in their lives. They reach a significant milestone at around second grade, when they begin to match events in their life with time on a clock. By adolescence, the basics of time management (telling time, understanding that tasks have deadlines, and understanding that task times vary) are well mastered. But keep in mind the caveat above about how many demands are imposed on teens today. You may not even have noticed much of a problem with your child's time management skills until he had a lot of options for how to spend his time and a lot of obligations to fulfill.

For adolescents, two key issues of time management are time planning and developing a sense of time urgency. Teens need to be adept at juggling options and obligations, preferred and less preferred or nonpreferred activities. The hallmark of a time management problem in a teen is underestimating how long it will take to do a nonpreferred task and overestimating how much time the teen has to complete that task. Related to this is a casual or relaxed approach and lack of a sense of urgency about approaching deadlines. Look more closely at your teen's management of time by filling out the questionnaire on the facing page. Feel free to photocopy it if you want to use the form more than once, such as for another teen.

Instilling Time Management in Everyday Situations

• *At least in matters involving your teen, try to ensure that you are modeling good time management practices.* If you are responsible for transportation to school, social events, or extracurricular activities, try to be on time. If you have made an arrangement to meet or complete an activity with your teen, make an effort to meet the time commitment. If your teen needs to talk with you and you cannot do it immediately, let her know when and for how long you will be available.

• *If you are following a routine or trying to get the teen to a scheduled event (such as giving your teen and her friends a ride), let her know how long it will take and when you need to leave to arrive on time.* Use calendars at home to mark

How Well Does Your Teen Manage Time?

For each item in the chart, first decide whether the statement to the left or right of *BUT* describes your teen better. Then rate the degree to which that statement applies to your teen. The number of items for which you chose the right-hand statement is an indicator of how much improvement your teen may need in the skill overall. Your ratings indicate possible targets for skill building: Where you chose "pretty much" or "very much" for a left-hand statement, your teen is demonstrating good use of the skill in that particular domain. "Pretty much" or "very much" for right-hand statements indicates areas that may need the most work.

Just a little	Pretty much	Very much				Just a little	Pretty much	Very much
			Some teens are always on time for school, dates, appointments, or other activities.	**BUT**	Other kids are chronically late.			
			Some kids are great at estimating how much time is needed to do something or go someplace.	**BUT**	Other kids have no idea how long it takes to do tasks or get from one place to another.			
			Some kids finish their homework or chores on time.	**BUT**	Other kids seem to routinely run out of time for things they need to do.			
			Some kids routinely accomplish the tasks they set out to do each day.	**BUT**	Other kids have difficulty doing everything they plan on getting done each day.			
			Some kids can adjust their pace to fit the time they have to finish something.	**BUT**	Other kids seem to work at one speed no matter how much time they will need to complete the task.			

family events and encourage your teen to use either paper calendars or planners, or calendars and alarms available on smartphones. At the time we are writing this, the latest version of smartphones allow voice-activated messages and alarms to be set for specific reminders, and these functions will certainly become increasingly sophisticated in the future.

• *Let your teen choose a timing device that will help him wake up and start his routine every morning.* This may be as simple as an alarm clock or as sophisticated as a smartphone application.

Managing Doctors' Appointments

Dr. Rasco (555-302-1024), make the appointment today, PLEASE!!! Marcia sighed and crumpled the Post-it note that was stuck to the phone in the kitchen.

"Robbie, did you call the doctor?"

Marcia already knew the answer to this question. She had purposely put the note over the keypad so Robbie would have to move it in order to make any call. She heard him thump down the stairs and looked over in time to see her energetic 15-year-old slide into the kitchen on his socks.

"What's up, Mom?"

She held up the phone. "Robbie, this is the third day in a row I have left you a note about calling the doctor. You are the one trying out for varsity soccer. You need to make an appointment for a physical because the school requires it if you are going to play."

Robbie scoffed, "Soccer tryouts? Mom, it's *June*."

Marcia mocked him lightly. "Robbie, it's the *end* of June. Tryouts are at the *end* of July, and practice starts at the *end* of August, so try to take this seriously and—"

"Okay, I know, I know. Gimme the phone. I'll call right now."

Robbie made a move out toward it, but Marcia backed it out of his reach. "No, they're closed now. We discussed this. It's why I leave a note for you, because before I leave and after I get home from work, the doctor's office is closed."

"Okay, Mom. Tomorrow I won't forget; I promise I'll call."

"Fine, good. Now, what would you like for dinner?"

The next morning before she left for work, Marcia made sure that Robbie wouldn't miss the reminders. She put Post-it notes on the phone, the counter, the coffeemaker, and the milk carton in the refrigerator. She put one on the mirror in the bathroom and one on the toilet seat. Finally, she went quietly into his room and put one on his soccer ball and one on the alarm clock. She leaned over, kissed her son good-bye, and left for work smiling. Everything would be fine, and this seemed like a good way to maintain a sense of humor while conveying to her son that the call needed to be made today.

When she came in that evening, Robbie was grumpy. "You didn't have to do that. I would have remembered—I would have. It seems like every time I forget something, you take over my memory. Every other step I took this morning, there was a Post-it note, smacking me in the face, telling me I'm bad at remembering."

Marcia felt hurt; that wasn't what she had meant by it at all, was it? It showed when she spoke. "I'm sorry. I didn't mean for it to look like that. It was supposed to be playful, a joke."

"Oh." His face softened immediately. "Well, I did call and make the appointment. July 20th at 3:00 P.M."

"Robbie, that's the day of tryouts."

"I know, it works out good. We just go there, then hop in the car and go to tryouts."

"Robbie, it's an hour before tryouts."

"And?"

"And the doctor's office is a half hour away."

"So? How long could a physical take?"

> As a kid, I'd put it off to the last second.
> —Matthew, age 18

"I don't know, Robbie, and that's the point. We really don't know how long we'll be there."

"I mean, worst-case scenario, I'll be like 5 or 10 minutes late."

"And that's the first impression you want to make? Robbie, why did you schedule them like this? The calendar was right on the fridge."

"You didn't tell me about that. You told me, 'Call the doctor and make an appointment.' You wrote it on a million frickin' Post-it notes, so that's what I did. They offered me a time, it fit, and I made the appointment."

"But the appointment might not fit, Robbie. You are constantly doing this. You can't make plans based on a theoretical timetable. Sure, the appointment's at three. But what if we're late, what if the doctor is, what if it takes a while, what if we get stuck in traffic on the way to tryouts?"

"What if a meteor hits the earth, Mom?"

"Enough! Go somewhere else. I'll deal with this."

"Whatever."

The next day, Marcia called the doctor's office to have the appointment changed, only to discover that all other available times before tryouts had been filled.

On the 20th, Marcia rushed home from work at 2:30 and found Robbie, still wet in a towel, running in circles, collecting cleats, shin guards, and socks that were stashed around the house.

"Sorry! Sorry, sorry, sorry. I thought I had time. I just got in the shower and kind of lost track of … of … Have you seen my cleat?"

"Cleats?"

"No, cleat. Just the left one."

"No, Robbie, I—" Marcia cut herself off. There would be no use arguing about it now. She ran around, found the other cleat in the garage, got Robbie into the car, and tore off to the doctor's office. Robbie was 15 minutes late for tryouts and was admonished by the coaches about first impressions.

That night, when his mother picked up Robbie from soccer practice, she said, "Robbie, this was a tough day for both of us. We were both stressed out, and your coaches weren't happy. Do you think we could work on a plan so that these kinds of situations go a little more smoothly?"

She and Robbie agreed to take some time on Saturday afternoon to talk more about the issue and try to work out an arrangement. Robbie indicated that even though he had not taken all of the issues into consideration, he did feel good about having made the appointment and agreed that he would be willing to take on more responsibility for appointments in the future. Thinking back to the situation, his mother realized that he did not have enough experience making appointments to take into consideration all the factors, such as commuting time, scheduling by others, and unanticipated delays. She and Robbie talked it over and decided that when it came to a particular appointment, they would discuss a list of items, including commuting time to and from the appointment, days that she and Robbie were available, building in enough time in case the appointment was a condition for an activity (like a sports physical), and building in "cushions" in case the person with whom the appointment was made was not on time. They also agreed that within a day of having this conversation Robbie would make the appointment. If his mother could be available, she would work through the issues when he was on the phone with the doctor's office, and if not, he would program a reminder in his phone, and with that as a backup she would also call him on the day he was supposed to make the appointment and give him a specific time to make the call.

> As a person who struggles with managing time myself, I would find such inflated times helpful. Organization and time management are quite linked, and helpful hints to both ends solve both problems.
>
> —Tasha, age 17

> *As Robbie, I would think it was important for my mother to help me. Overall what she did for him seemed reasonable, but over time I would let Robbie do more on his own.*
> —Lorie, age 16

Over the next 2 months, Robbie was able to schedule a dental checkup and a follow-up appointment to have a filling.

In late October, Marcia drove to the field behind the school at 5:30 P.M. Robbie was sitting on the bleachers with his socks pulled down and his shin guards flapping around his ankles. When he saw his mother, he yanked up his cleats, socks, and guards and threw them all in a gym bag, out of which he pulled a pair of flip-flops.

> *I would be appreciative of the help, but probably a bit miffed at first.*
> —Tasha, age 17

"I see you are fully equipped today."

"And on time!"

> *It is critical that kids get in the habit of planning "cushion time."*
> —Ben, age 17

"I just want to say you've done a good job, Robbie. You handled the dentist appointments and, as far as soccer goes, changing at the field was a great idea for keeping your things from being strewn around the house."

"And the coach took my recommendation and started a Facebook group for the team, and now he posts a calendar and lists games and events so we can both keep track of what things are coming up."

> *I think the mom should have had more faith and understanding in Robbie and Robbie more patience. I think that the Saturday talk was a good idea and they will see results from that.*
> —Teo, age 15

Q & A

Like Robbie, with a lot of coaching and practice and some teen-friendly tools, my son eventually learned to make appointments and to remind himself that they were coming up. But after all that planning, he still seems to be late about half of the time because he doesn't allow enough time to get there. What's going on?

Ninety-nine percent of the time, a teen with a time management issue will under- rather than overestimate the length of time something will take. You may be thinking that we all do this here and there, and that's absolutely true. With your teen, though, this is often the result of oversimplifying the situation.

If a teen with these problems knows that a doctor's appointment is supposed to be a half hour long and that the doctor's office is 15 minutes away, this information might lead the teen to conclude that the entire round-trip process will take one hour. So the teen waits until 2 minutes before that hour begins to leave, only to discover his or her car keys are nowhere to be found. The teen's time estimate will neglect to allow for unforeseen circumstances, and this is what usually gets him into trouble. We've seen teenagers allow exactly the amount of travel time that a trip should take under ideal circumstances even when they live in a city that often suffers gridlock, when they live in a rural area that has volatile, traffic-impeding weather, or when they know their car sometimes balks at starting up right away.

So what can you do? We recommend that teens like Robbie and your son set the clocks on personal devices ahead of the actual time. We understand that this request might be greeted with a chortle from your teen, "Obviously I'll know that it's not the *real* time." You can explain to your teen that the intent isn't ultimately to fool him into thinking it is a different time. The point is to get him to take action as if it is the correct time. Odds are that if he does this he will sometimes arrive at appointments early, but sometimes he will be right on time due to unforeseen delays. The goal is for these accumulated experiences to serve as a reminder of how important it is to allow extra time for those unexpected events.

My daughter says I never say anything in 5 words if I can say it in 50. So I've tried really hard to keep my reminders and instructions brief. But now she takes me so literally that when she finally does what I've asked she does it without regard for any other considerations that I haven't stated explicitly. I posted a bunch of reminders Saturday morning for her to walk the dog. We were going to a family reunion that evening and would be gone for hours, and last time we had an event like that she spent too much time on everything she wanted to get done before going out, and the dog didn't get a walk. We found a big mess when we got home. This time I thought the reminders would do the trick, but she walked the dog first thing in the morning—"so I'd have time," as she explained. What else can I do?

For teens like Robbie and your daughter, expect vague directions to be followed vaguely. It may be obvious to you that if you're going out at night and will be gone for hours, the dog needs to be walked right before you leave. It may have been obvious to Marcia that Robbie needed to take into account the tryout schedule, the travel time to and from the doctor's office, and everything else that most adults consider when scheduling an event. So the Post-its Marcia left and the conversation she had with him told Robbie only that he needed to make an appointment as soon as possible. Kids with time management problems will often focus only on their specific task, which would be a good thing if they had previously consulted a schedule or calendar to make sure that nothing else interfered with it. In this case Robbie did that, but his inability to add up the time the whole appointment could take—travel time to and from, a potentially backed-up doctor's schedule, the exam itself—and how that would fit with the scheduled time for the tryouts kept him from making the appointment for a time that would work for him. Again, teens with time management problems may tend to cement ill-conceived timetables in their heads. For Robbie, June is the beginning of summer and there are months and months (in reality there are two) until the fall school year. In his mind, the first day of school is in September, so school-related obligations start then. It is important to impart to these teens that events are more fluid than that, undulating or going from priority to back burner, but they never disappear. Your daughter probably never thought about how long the dog would be stuck in the house, and therefore it didn't occur to her that it would be wise to walk the dog right before leaving. Your option could have been to say not just "Don't forget to walk the dog" but "Please walk the dog between 4:00 and 5:00 today." When the factors involved may be more complicated, as they were for Robbie's doctor's appointment, writing them down, or better yet texting them, is the best idea. Or have the teen get in the habit (by including it in the text or even standing there while the teen does it if necessary) of creating an event in the teen's cell phone calendar, so the phone alarm would sound at 4:15 with an accompanying text message that says "Time to walk the dog!"

18

Encouraging Goal-Directed Persistence

Goal-directed persistence involves the capacity to establish a goal and follow through on achieving it without being put off or distracted by competing interests. The couple that wants to buy a house and is saving money for the down payment demonstrates goal-directed persistence. The 11-year-old who spends hours every week practicing ball handling and shooting baskets to make the basketball team shows goal-directed persistence. The 16-year-old who gets a job and puts her money away to eventually buy a car evidences goal-directed persistence. To reach a goal, you must appreciate the fact that your day-in and day-out behavior has a direct impact on whether you will get there.

How Goal-Directed Persistence Develops

Goal-directed persistence is one of the last executive skills to mature fully, sometime in the early to mid-20s for most young adults. This, naturally, does not stop us from encouraging our children to develop the skill throughout childhood and adolescence. We might start by guiding our toddler to assemble a puzzle or helping our 5-year-old master bike riding. From an early age, we encourage our children to persist and try to impress upon them the fact that mastering new skills will take practice, repetition, time, and effort. Our children are exposed to the notion of persistence in different aspects of their lives—playing sports, learning to read or do math, playing a musical instrument, and doing household chores. When younger, we encouraged them to work at their goals for brief periods of time, gradually increasing the time as they got older and their skills developed. We also probably helped them set up a plan to save money to buy a desired item.

By the time they enter high school, most teens have had the experience of having to practice a skill, save money, or work at a task to achieve a goal. But how successfully have they done this? Adolescence can impact goal-directed persistence by offering teens a lot more choices for how to spend their time (and money) than they had when younger. Now they may prefer to hang out with friends instead of researching colleges. Now they might pay for a pizza and a movie for themselves and a date instead of putting that money aside for the new mountain bike they want. Now they might have goals that conflict with your goals for them, and they will probably start arguing for their right to set their own priorities.

If your teen is weak in goal-directed persistence, context-dependent behavior (see Chapters 1 and 5) may have an even more potent pull on him. As Russell Barkley has noted, teens who lag behind in this executive skill are much more likely to focus their attention on the current situation than on how their behavior might impact their future goal. Let's say your teen expresses a desire to go to a particular college and understands that that means getting a certain grade-point average, which in turn means getting assignments in on time and studying for tests. The teen who is context dependent might intend to study on Sunday for a Monday test but would be likely to opt for the immediate gratification of going to Facebook, going out to meet friends, or watching a favorite TV show. If he can't resist the pull or temptation of the immediate situation and does not connect his current behavior with future goals, goal-directed persistence will be a problem for the teen and for you.

Take a closer look at your teen's ability to persist at reaching a goal by completing the questionnaire on page 234. Feel free to photocopy it if you want to use the form more than once, such as for another teen.

Increasing Goal-Directed Persistence from Day to Day

• *Whenever possible, work on persistence toward a goal that your teen has an investment in.* Doing this demonstrates respect for your teen's desire to be independent and make her own decisions and gives you a built-in motivator. Sometimes her goals and your goals for her will coincide and there is no conflict. If you agree on one of her goals (for example, getting a car), negotiate the

How Well Does Your Teen Persist toward a Goal?

For each item in the chart, first decide whether the statement to the left or right of *BUT* describes your teen better. Then rate the degree to which that statement applies to your teen. The number of items for which you chose the right-hand statement is an indicator of how much improvement your teen may need in the skill overall. Your ratings indicate possible targets for skill building: Where you chose "pretty much" or "very much" for a left-hand statement, your teen is demonstrating good use of the skill in that particular domain. "Pretty much" or "very much" for right-hand statements indicates areas that may need the most work.

Just a little	Pretty much	Very much				Just a little	Pretty much	Very much
			Some kids have one eye on the future and how best to get there.	BUT	Other kids prefer to take one day at a time.			
			Some kids are willing to set aside fun stuff to achieve long-term goals.	BUT	Other kids live by the motto "You're only young once."			
			Some kids know what they want to do when they grow up and have a plan for getting there.	BUT	Other kids don't think about life after high school or college but assume they will know what they want to do "when the time comes."			
			Some kids set goals and don't let anything stop them from reaching their goals.	BUT	Other kids see what is happening right now as more important than what is down the road.			
			Some kids don't let obstacles stand in the way of getting what they want.	BUT	Other kids give up working toward a goal if something blocks them.			

particulars with your teen, but do not compromise on critical issues such as safety.

• *If your teen has goals that you can agree to, but you have conditions or expectations surrounding the goal, be sure to let him know specifically what these are in advance.* For example, if your teen is interested in a particular college, let him know what limitations you need him to keep in mind, such as cost or location. For car purchases, in addition to cost, this could include safety features, repair considerations, and so forth. By giving the teen certain limits that he needs to take into consideration, you help him refine the process of goal-directed behavior.

> *It is hard to go after what you want when you don't know where to start or even when you don't know what you want, and kids struggle with these things. Motivation is the difference maker when it comes to goal-directed persistence in teenagers most of the time, in my opinion.*
> —Ben, age 17

• *If the goal your teen sets is well into the future, help her set some concrete benchmarks along the way so that she can have the sense that she is making progress toward her goal.* In the case of saving money for some goal, this might be reflected in maintaining some sort of passbook savings account or regularly reviewing an online account. In the case of preparing for college, ongoing monitoring of grades and matching these against college requirements would have this effect.

• *Maintain interest in longer-term goals by keeping them visible and concrete.* This might involve making online or in-person visits to colleges, meeting with college representatives, and gathering information and materials. In the case of purchases (cars, phones, etc.), this would mean periodically searching what's out there and looking for updates. In Chapter 7, we listed various steps that teens could follow to reach a particular goal.

• *For goals you care about but your teen does not, use an incentive to help the teen stick with it.* See Chapter 5 for more details on incentives. Basically, however, you need to think about whether the goal is short- or long-term. If long-term—for example, maintaining decent grades—you'll likely need to have ongoing incentives to help your teen stay focused. If there are shorter-term tasks, such as studying for specific tests or completion of chores, the use of a "first–then" system is most effective: the less preferred task (for example, studying) must be completed before the teen engages in a more preferred task of her choice (for example, going out with friends or playing a video game). When your teen is more context dependent than goal directed, you will win her attention and spur immediate motivation—that is, change the context—by providing access to something she wants and finds rewarding. Above all, remain positive with your teen. A good attitude can transform ordering your teen to do something into encouraging her to develop responsible habits that will lead to greater independence in the future.

Desire Alone Does Not Always Produce a Result: Helping a Teen Achieve His Goal

"Do you think it's hard to get tickets? Maya says it's almost impossible, but I think that's just an excuse for her not to go to the games. She thinks football is boring."

"She's not alone," Dante's mother chimed in from her office off the living room, where Dante and his dad were watching college football. Dante's older sister attended one of the schools playing in the game, and Dante hoped to go to the same school when he graduated.

"I don't think she has very much time," said Dante's dad. "From what I hear, she's buried in her books most of the time. The workload there is demanding, especially when you think of the courses she's taking."

"Speaking of books," said Dante's mother, "when are you going to crack open the ones we brought you, Dante? You've been talking about this for some time, and yet they're still in the shrink wrap they came in."

Dante had decided, practically the day after his sister was accepted, that he wanted to go to the college she was attending. His sister was bright and had handled high school easily, while Dante could lag behind without proper rein-forcement. Sometimes Dante's parents felt he was adrift: willing to be pushed by waves of encouragement and pressure but lacking a constant current to drive him toward his goals. Sometimes he chose to pursue something without really considering what it took to achieve it. For instance, last year he had decided he wanted to learn the piano. His parents happily found him a teacher, but because Dante did not practice regularly, he never progressed at the rate he expected to, and his playing languished. At times it seemed like an unfortunate cycle: Dante was bright and wanted to be good at things, but his failure to stick with them on a day-to-day basis meant he rarely met his own expectations and subsequently abandoned his goals. This had happened thus far with only minor consequences, but Dante's parents knew that if he followed this pattern with his goal of getting into his sister's competitive school, the results could be devastating for everyone.

"I'll get to the books, I really will."

And he did, at first, but Dante's studying became uncoordinated and erratic. His parents reminded him again of his goals, and for a few days he put in a lot of effort to cover the material in the test-prep books. Again this pace proved unsustainable, and his efforts dropped off after a week. Dante's parents knew they could remind him constantly about studying for the tests, but they were worried for a couple of reasons: (1) they could help him through this stage, but if he got into the school, they wouldn't be able to help him there; and (2) they had tried this before, and it resulted in frequent arguments between Dante and them over issues of irresponsibility and independence.

A few months later, Dante came home to find a letter for him from the testing board. He opened it and discovered that he had scored well below what he would need to be considered a competitive candidate at his sister's school. Dante was dejected; he recalled having studied quite a bit for these tests. Why the bad scores?

Later that night, Dante and his parents had a sit-down discussion at the table.

"Dante," his mother started out, "we know how badly you want to go to the same college as Maya. We want you to as well. But you need to understand that even Maya didn't get there without persistent hard work. She studied on a schedule; she took practice tests seriously and frequently. Call her; talk to her about it. We can help you set up a schedule and give you reminders if that's what you want. But the primary mover and shaker here is you, Dante. There's no way around it."

Dante nodded, and they began to devise a plan. He called his sister, who gave him a rundown of her study schedule and some helpful hints. From then until the next time he took the test, Dante had an "appointment" with his test-prep books for 20 minutes each weekday. He took a practice test every other week. Although his parents reminded him of things here and there, he relied primarily on the alarm function of his cell phone, programming in daily and weekly alarms signaling his study times. Even after the routine had sunk in, he kept the alarms going because they made sure he kept up his pace. For Dante, it wasn't about just performing a task; it was about being constantly reminded that it was there, day after day, to the point where it

> *Alarms accomplish the goal of turning motivation into action.*
> Tasha, age 17

stopped being something he either wanted or didn't want, liked or didn't like, and simply became something that was done, as regular as brushing his teeth.

We have tried reminders and alarms without success. What's going on in Dante's situation that makes it different?

There has to be motivation and a plan behind the action. Alarm clocks and cell phones can be good signaling devices, and setting reminders is fine, but without a corresponding reinforcement of the ultimate goal behind these daily cues, they become a nuisance rather than a motivator. Like it or not, we as parents are frequently the mouthpieces of goal-directed persistence when it comes to our children. For your teen to develop a sense of independence and learn to motivate himself, this idea of investment must be transferred from you to your child. It is not supposed to be about what Dante's parents want; it's about his desire to go to his sister's college. Teens going through this transitional period in their lives are forming their ideas about themselves. Part of this involves extricating themselves from the aspirations their parents have for them and deciding for themselves which ones they want.

Another factor that may be at work here is anxiety on your teen's part about her executive skills weaknesses. She may be well aware that she struggles in areas that other students excel in, seemingly without any pressure or difficulty. But what your teen needs to understand is that alarm cues and reminders are not just crutches used by people with a weakness in goal-directed persistence; they are also the hallmarks of people who welcome and effectively employ time management in conjunction with an understanding that daily work is the foundation of long-term success and goal achievement. So we certainly would advocate that parents look beyond their own anecdotes and experiences to find peers who exhibit these qualities. Showing Dante through these examples that there is no shame and much success and gratification to be found in employing these techniques may make him more apt to adopt them into his own routines. In Dante's situation, his parents might want to reach out to his sister and have her let Dante know that her success wasn't some magical secret and give him some strategies that she used. If you notice a friend of your teen's who has particularly good skills, encourage your teen to consult with him or her, even if just casually. Sometimes teens like Dante might be self-conscious about asking peers for help, but even observation or offhand remarks might lend insight into how their peers function effectively, without openly revealing your teen's problem. Another way might be to relate persistence to a subject your teen likes, such as sports. Good athletes say that practice always trumps natural ability in when it comes to attaining success in their sport. In the same way, your teen may not be born with great organizational skills, but that isn't as big a determining factor as daily reinforcement of good habits.

My teen has very similar difficulties sticking to a routine. She is adamant about the goal she is trying to reach, but after a few days or weeks the effort level drops considerably, and I find myself back where I started, cajoling her into doing tasks and creating tension between us.

The most important piece of advice we can offer is this: *Teach your child to respect the sanctity of the routine.* Consistency in the repetition of the task is critical to long-term success. A strict routine needs to be put in place, so ideally, if the task involves something like studying for an entrance exam, it would be performed at the same pace at the same time every day, or on certain days of the week, every week. If this level of consistency is not possible, then consider having a study period that piggybacks onto some regular event or activity. If the family eats dinner together, perhaps there is a time slot available before or afterward. If your teen has a particular television show or a time at which she regularly watches shows, encourage her to do her studying right before that. It helps if there is a specific time and space for the study routine. Bookending the activity will help alleviate the sense that something tedious is lasting forever.

Another tip: Be positive! Your teen wants things for herself, and that is an important first step. Hounding her in a negative manner when the routine slips is counterproductive; it shifts the focus from achieving the goal to not satisfactorily meeting your expectations. This will land you in a fight and may sour her on the activity in general, so if your teen falters, approach her as calmly and positively as possible. Make sure to keep the focus on the fact that this is something she wants for herself. Encourage her to include messages and cell phone reminders that reinforce the long-term goal. If studying is involved, suggest that your teen track her progress visually. This could be as simple as putting checkmarks next to the material that has been covered in the table of contents of a test prep book. Finally, in the case of SATs or ACTs, the teen needs to do the practice tests! Familiarity and comfort with test content is a big leg up, and nothing validates those hours of studying like regularly improving scores.

19

....

Cultivating Metacognition

Metacognition refers to the ability to stand back and observe yourself from the outside—how you problem-solve and what is called for in a given situation. When you have this skill, you can factor multiple sources of information into your decisions about how to proceed in the circumstances before you, based on what you understand about yourself. While you are proceeding, you can also monitor and evaluate your own behavior, asking yourself, "How am I doing?" Afterward, you can also evaluate how you did and then decide whether to do things differently in the future based on that evaluation. Metacognition is a skill that is based on a combination of understanding your own behavior and past experiences and monitoring your behavior as you adjust to some current situation. People who lack this skill have difficulty making use of their own observations and of feedback from others to correct their behavior for the future. For example, a teen who was previously let go from a job for not showing "initiative" gets another job in a supermarket. When he is not given a specific job by his manager, he spends time texting friends rather than using free time to stock shelves. A girl has an argument with her best friend and later that night posts negative comments about her on Facebook even though doing that had ended another friendship that she valued in the past.

How Metacognition Develops

We see the earliest examples of metacognition in young children when they solve a problem or use a strategy. For example, a young child might make an adjustment in putting a puzzle together when his first attempt fails or when he

240

makes a suggestion to another child for how to solve a problem. The seven- or eight-year-old can adjust her behavior in response to feedback from a teacher or parent, or, when observing what happens to others, can change behavior appropriately. In these examples, children demonstrate strategy use, but it is not metacognition as we think of it in the adolescent or adult sense because they do not step back and observe themselves and think in advance about strategy use. At around eleven years old, children can begin to anticipate the consequence of a course of action and make adjustments or propose several solutions to a problem and explain which one might be best. By late middle to early high school, the teen can evaluate her own performance on a school assignment or in a sports event or see the impact of her behavior on peers and make adjustments. Thus, in adolescence, when given feedback, teens can "look" at themselves and adjust their behavior when they have metacognitive skills. Weaknesses in metacognitive skills are manifested by a seeming inability to learn from one's mistakes and profit from experience. When parents witness weak metacognitive skills in their teen, they ask, "When are you going to realize that if you continue to do this you're going to [lose your license, have no friends, get fired, etc.]?" Get a better idea of your teen's metacognitive skills by using the questionnaire on page 242. Feel free to photocopy it if you want to use the form more than once, such as for another teen.

Improving Metacognitive Skills in Your Teen's Life

• *Provide specific praise for key elements of task performance by recognizing strategies that your teen uses.* For instance, say to your teen "You're good at understanding your friends' feelings" or "I admire the way you take your coach's feedback and convert it to an action." To do this, you need to look for examples of chores at home, performance on school assignments, and interactions with friends to see when your teen uses problem-solving strategies or can accept feedback from others and change his behavior.

• *Encourage your teen to evaluate her own performance on a task or in a social situation.* With teens, this can be a delicate enterprise and is better managed by questions than statements. For example, if your teen tells you that a friend said something hurtful to her, suggesting or even implying that she may have done something to trigger this is likely to provoke a defensive response. You might instead ask her to tell you about the interaction and then ask if she can see anything in the interaction that might have triggered the hurtful comment.

How Well Does Your Teen Use Metacognitive Skills?

For each item in the chart, first decide whether the statement to the left or right of *BUT* describes your teen better. Then rate the degree to which that statement applies to your teen. The number of items for which you chose the right-hand statement is an indicator of how much improvement your teen may need in the skill overall. Your ratings indicate possible targets for skill building: Where you chose "pretty much" or "very much" for a left-hand statement, your teen is demonstrating good use of the skill in that particular domain. "Pretty much" or "very much" for right-hand statements indicates areas that may need the most work.

Just a little	Pretty much	Very much				Just a little	Pretty much	Very much
			Some kids are good at stepping back and seeing the "whole picture."	BUT	Other kids get lost in details and miss this big picture.			
			Some kids are good at sensing how others are reacting to their behavior or ideas.	BUT	Other kids focus more on getting their point across and may not pick up on feedback from others.			
			Some kids try to figure out what went wrong so they can do better the next time.	BUT	Other kids put their mistakes behind them and hope they do not happen again.			
			Some kids can come up with several different ways to study.	BUT	Other kids have only one way to study, and it does not always work.			
			Some kids ask for feedback from teachers or coaches to help them improve performance.	BUT	Other kids don't even think about asking for feedback and just assume they know what they are doing.			

Another approach is to frame it by recognizing that the teen has a strength first. For example, you might say something like "You're a confident person, and I wonder if your friend's reaction came because he felt insecure in this situation." This may or may not lead to insight on the teen's part, but it is likely to open up the possibility of more discussion rather than triggering a defensive reaction.

• *Encourage the teen to ask for performance evaluations as a way to improve his performance.* For example, suggest that the teen approach teachers or bosses with the statement "I'd like to do better on _____. Are there some specific things that I could do to improve?" While this is an effective strategy with which to approach teachers or supervisors, if a person in a position of authority is already frustrated with the teen, he may not respond in a constructive way.

• *Use your behavior as a way of indirectly helping your teen understand how people might react to her behavior.* For example, telling your teen how your tone of voice or body posture is interpreted by other people and even giving her an example may help her appreciate this behavior in herself, as long as she does not perceive it as a lecture or as fault finding directed toward her.

> Sometimes adults have a hard time looking in the mirror. While these problems are prevalent in adolescence, adults are not above them.
> —Tasha, age 17

• *In situations where your interaction with the teen is a source of conflict, and you feel that he is reacting to a behavior that you both bring to the situation (for example, an angry tone of voice), go to your teen at a "neutral" time and talk about* **your** *behavior and your reaction to the situation.* For example, "Devlin, when we talked about _____ the other day, I got angry and raised my voice. I'm going to do my best to stay calm when we talk about these things in the future." In this situation, you use your own behavior as a model for how you would like your teen to adjust his behavior. Your calm tone of voice makes it more likely that he will be calm (remember "hot" versus "cool" cognition). If you notice that your teen is making an attempt to be calm, you can comment on the positive change in the discussion: "Thanks for helping me with this. I really appreciate it when we can talk calmly."

Learning to Listen to Feedback

Aina came home from school on Tuesday and dropped her bag inside the door. She felt tired and disappointed. She unzipped the bag and took out a binder that had most of her loose work in it. Opening the binder on the coffee table, Aina took out her most recent English assignment, a five-page book report on *Jane Eyre*. Aina scratched the red C– in the top left corner with her thumbnail. *Sure, I didn't give a lot of time and brain juice to this paper, but a C–?* She flipped to the last page, where her teacher had jotted comments. Aina rarely read the teacher's comments on major assignments; she simply looked at the grade and saw "looks good" or "do better work," but she was confused by this low grade. As soon as she saw that the comments began, "Solid thesis, but paragraphs were loose and grammar problems abound"—she stopped reading.

Paragraphs were loose? That doesn't even mean anything, and my grammar was fine; I'm sure of that. True, at the time she was writing, Aina did think the paper was grammatically sound, but Aina is not in the habit of revising and proofreading her work. She meant what she wrote when she wrote it. Generally, her grammar is a nonissue, but Aina wrote this paper at the last minute, and a number of errors slipped in due to the pressure.

Aina went to the refrigerator and grabbed a seltzer water. When she closed the door, she noticed the A history paper attached to it that she had written a year ago. She had not had one since, and Aina really couldn't see why. She felt like the same writer. She read her writing and thought she saw similar patterns in all of it.

Aina showed the paper to her mother later that night. Mom had helped her in the past when there were things wrong with her writing.

"So I really didn't see anything wrong with it. Looks pretty much like all the other B work I've done."

"Well, in some cases, 'pretty much like' and 'exactly like' can be a difference between a C– and a B, Aina. Did you look at her corrections and comments?"

"Kind of. She said something about grammar and loose paragraphs. I didn't see it."

"Well, the grammar stuff is pretty evident. These pages are pecked all over with red ink. Look here: *true creative is original*. You see that, Aina? I mean, no noun to speak of, and originality is implicit in the definition of creativity, don't you think? It reads like a bad line from a car commercial; you're better than that. *True creative is original, original beautiful is inspirational, inspirational is creative, creative is true* . . . " Aina's mom fell over sideways on the couch, laughing. Aina feigned annoyance.

"Yeah, yeah, okay. I get it. But seriously, though, I remember getting A's all the time for work exactly like this, just a little cleaner. What's changed?"

"Well, maybe it would pay to sit down and ask yourself that very question. What has changed? You're in a new grade, taking different classes with new teachers. Have you thought about what their expectations are, or that your work is expected to progress as you get older? The same things that worked once aren't always going to. You have to think about how you approach things, what strategies work and which ones don't, what your strengths and weaknesses are, how you highlight the former and shore up the latter."

"Yeah, I kind of see where you're going with that."

"For instance, you're a junior now, Aina. Teachers are not going to tolerate rampant grammatical errors in major assignments. Maybe you weren't called out on it as much last year because it was a more forgivable offense. Did you consider this?"

> I feel like the story with Aina does not make her any better at seeing faults in herself, just better at fixing the faults her parents point out to her. The solution to Aina's problem did not solve her metacognitive failures, but it helped her get the grade for her class.
> —Tasha, age 17

"No, I never thought about it that way. It does kind of make sense, though."

"Well, maybe we could sit down tomorrow and start to brainstorm some ideas about how we can update how you analyze these factors. Sound good?"

"I think you meant, 'Does that sound like a good idea to you, Aina?' You know, noun, verb, subject, object, et cetera."

"Hahaha, okay, I get it."

Q & A

That vignette helps us understand metacognition in this situation, but we're the ones who have to have tomorrow's conversation, too. How do we explain metacognition to our teens and suggest ways to develop it?

Maybe the simpler way for your teen to understand metacognition is the phrase "third-person thinking." Of course, "third person" is a term that has its history in narrative, but most teens will associate it with video games. A third-person video game is one in which the user can see the entire character he is using, controlling its interactions with the environment. Similarly, metacognition is about taking a bird's-eye view of one's own thought process—thinking about thinking.

Going back to the idea of narrative and writing, we would like to suggest a metaphor that might help your teen understand metacognition. Imagine for a second that our thought processes are one long continuous paper being typed in our heads. We do not need to go and revise it because we are writing (or thinking, in this case) about things we are very familiar with. Driving, brushing teeth, cooking (well, for some of us), and other routine activities are not things we really think hard about doing. But, if we are doing our taxes or an important piece of work or literally writing a paper, we routinely go back to reread and edit what we have written (or thought). In the same way, when we plan something important in our heads or prepare to perform a complex task, we, using meta-cognition, go back and "edit" our thoughts to make sure that they are in sync with what is required for the situation.

Now, when we are writing things like informal e-mails, Facebook status updates, tweets, or scribbled notes, we rarely go over them with a fine-toothed grammatical comb; we save this kind of scrutiny for in-depth, consequential work. But imagine if this system was faulty, if when we wrote a paper we treated it as if it were an e-mail we put aside the idea of careful conception and just wrote. The paper would probably be a mess, right?

Well, teens with metacognition problems have this type of difficulty, except it is expanded to include not just major assignments but any complicated task in life. They may also have diminished overall ability and therefore not be able to apply metacognition to things others might consider routine. Broken down, developing metacognition is about employing a look-before-you-leap philoso-phy based on past experience and/or feedback from other people. Your teen, like Aina, is probably not considering all the angles when he does something. This is a difficult skill because it requires flexibility; metacognition starts with a recognition that the games and rules are subject to change. If you understand how you play the game, you will be better able to adjust to situations when the rules change.

Metacognition and impulsivity are addressed separately in this book, but the two often seem like the same problem. How are they different and how can we as parents tell the difference between the two? If our teen is weak in both, how can we dif-ferentiate between what is a metacognition problem and what is an impulse control problem?

We agree wholeheartedly with the statement above. Behaviorally, metacogni-tion and impulse control problems will manifest in very similar ways, especially if they co-occur. But they are neurologically distinct skills that happen when either function is being used. Response inhibition is characterized by the abil-ity to delay what would otherwise be an immediate act. Time delay is the key. In many situations, your teen must have the skill of response inhibition to use metacognition. But simply delaying a response doesn't mean that you have good metacognition. Metacognition requires that you stand back and "see" yourself in a situation and, based on past experience and knowledge about yourself, use this information to decide what works and what doesn't in the current situation. In the examples earlier about the boy in the grocery store or the girl posting on Facebook, impulsivity wasn't the problem. Neither of them used past experience to avoid making the same mistake. Metacognition is at work when one looks at a problem and can (1) articulate several possible solutions and (2) identify which solution is best and why. Measured self-reflection and self-analysis are also a part of metacognition; one is able to rate past actions and performances and put them to work in such a way that they inform future behavior.

Pizza

Tuesday night was all-you-can-eat pizza night at Gigi's, and for Matt and his friends it was as ingrained a tradition as 16-year-olds can have. John was the first one to get his license, in December, and every Tuesday since then he had picked the rest of them up at the public basketball court that was the epicenter of their respective neighborhoods. All the boys loved these nights because they were always lively and occasionally raucous, and they were the teens' first unsupervised public outings.

Out of the entire crew, Matt was the one who tended to push the envelope the most. It might start with an eating or chugging contest and some light verbal jousting. But often Matt would find himself caught up in a level of revelry that was degrees beyond his friends. He might steal others' pizza, loosen the top of the salt shaker so when someone used it he dumped salt all over himself, or peel back someone's cheese with a fork and mix red pepper flakes and Tabasco in with the pizza sauce while the other person was in the bathroom. While initially met with laughter and general goodwill, these antics grew stale with repetition. Most people would have simply moved on. But Matt often missed cues telling him that things were beginning to sour. In fact, if he felt that he wasn't getting the laughs he wanted, he often upped the ante, pulling more and more outrageous stunts under the assumption that the greater the prank, the greater the response.

The second Tuesday in March, Matt jogged up to Tim and Steve, who were lobbing a tennis ball against one of the backboards. "Hey, where's Evan?" Matt asked.

"Dunno," said Steve. "He texted Tim and said he wasn't coming, said he had something to do. Maybe he doesn't want to get pantsed again like you did to him last week."

"Oh, whatever," Matt said. "I didn't even really do it, not that I could, his belt was cinched like he knew it was coming. And that was after he hit me with a snowball anyway. He's just being soft."

"S'pose so," said Tim, laughing softly.

They went to Gigi's that night, and although Matt did his best, the mood wasn't quite as elevated as before. Jokes that had gotten laughs before got chuckles. The salt shaker prank got only a sigh from Tim, who got up, threw the whole thing in the trash, and got another slice, this time sitting down a seat farther away from Matt. Usually they would retaliate, but tonight they just seemed exasperated. Matt gave it his all, did his best to put his friends in a better mood, but it was to no avail, and the ride home was quiet.

The next week Matt walked to the basketball court, but no one else was there. He waited for 5, 10, 15 minutes and then, seeing no one, turned and went home. The next day at school, he saw Tim and caught up to him in the hallway.

"Hey, man!"

"Oh, hey, Matt, what's going on?"

Matt eyed him, "What happened to you guys last night? I waited at the court for a while."

Tim laughed. "Oh, sorry, man, I don't know what happened. John said he'd pick us up at the school because he and Steve had to stay after for detention. One of them was supposed to text you. Ask them—maybe they spaced or thought they already told you."

Mark found John, Evan, and Steve throughout the day and asked them what had happened. Each one gave him the same story, saying that he thought one of the others had texted him and just figured he was doing something else. Matt laughed it off and went home.

That night when he sat down for dinner, Mark's parents asked him if he had figured out what happened.

"Yeah, the guys just had a miscommunication. Each one of them said they thought one of the others had texted me, and when I didn't respond they thought I was busy."

Matt's father put his fork down and looked over. "Does that really make sense to you, Matt?"

"I mean, yeah. Why, should it not?"

His mother spoke, "Matt, you and your friends have been going to Tuesday night pizza, without fail, for the better part of 4 months. Now all of a sudden they all make it there without trying to contact you more diligently than just assuming the others had taken care of it?"

Matt looked confused. "Matt," his dad said, "what your mother is saying is that . . . isn't it possible that your friends left you out? Maybe the reason they 'forgot' was that they didn't want you to go this time?"

Matt pondered this, and as he did his confusion turned to anger, and soon he was seething.

"Wait, Matt," his mother said as she put her hand over his. "Before you get mad, think about why they might have done this. It doesn't make sense that they would just all of a sudden cut you out for no reason. Maybe forgetting about you wasn't an ethically sound thing to do. But often those kinds of actions come from a desire to be discreet. Maybe you offended them, and instead of confronting you they decided to 'accidentally' leave you behind. Is there anything you can think of that would make them want to do this?"

Matt thought for a while and then told them about the pizza pranks and the joking that went on. He mentioned Evan's absence 2 weeks prior and related the offhand remarks from the others about what might have kept him from coming. His parents nodded.

"So, Matt, isn't it feasible that you were going overboard with everything and they just got tired of it?," asked Matt's father. "It's not bullying, because there isn't malicious intent, but more that you lack a sense of how others are reacting to you or have in the past? This may have been building up for some time, but overall your friends tolerate it because they like you. Then one week Evan breaks the cipher by leaving, and that becomes a catalyst for everyone else, who follow suit by quietly, and without telling you why outright, cut you from Tuesday night pizza."

> *I would say it's common for self-review of actions to be influenced by what others think. The need for acceptance can lead teens not to care about themselves as long as they are widely accepted by peers. Self-review is guided by what the crowd is doing during the teen years, and resulting adjustments from self-review are as well.*
>
> —Ben, age 17

"So—so now what?" Matt asked. "What do you think I should do?"

"Well, it certainly seems like you may have gone overboard. You know as well as anyone else, Matt, that when you tell the same joke over and over, it loses its oomph. It sounds like pizza night for your friends has come to signify, to some degree, you making one big long joke, the same joke, week after week. So I would say the best thing to do would be to apologize, without acknowledging that their forgetting you might have been intentional; that part isn't important. Then wait and see if you get invited next week. If you don't, then your mother or I can drive you there to meet them. Either way, once you get there, step off the gas pedal for a while. Humor can be spectacle, but among close friends, more often than not, it is intimate and reaffirms the friendships rather than singling out people for humiliation. A few well-placed remarks will take you further than pantsing someone or ruining his food. Remember that, and keep in mind past reactions of friends to your antics; if there is something that makes them upset, avoid it. Think about what else is going on before you act."

"In short," his mother quipped, "if you get too saucy, you'll become cheesy. And if you keep roasting your friends, they'll get burnt out, and then all you'll be is left over."

"Mom!" Matt feigned annoyance, "Okay . . . I'll admit, that was actually pretty solid. Thanks for the advice, guys."

20

···

Coaching

Throughout this book we have included school performance problems that illustrate the effects of executive skills weaknesses in teenagers and how they can be addressed. As you know, delays in the development of various executive skills can affect your teenager in every domain of life, but it's academics that may very well cause you the most concern. That's understandable: achievement in school represents a key to your teen's future, including the ability to earn a decent living, live independently, and attain career satisfaction. Unfortunately, school performance problems also can be a source of significant conflict between parents and teens. If you've been closely monitoring your child's schoolwork since elementary or middle school, those efforts may now feel like babying to your teen. If you've been collaborating with your teen's teachers for years to help him keep up, having regular contact with his high school teachers may be seen as meddling. You may believe that cutting off all of these supports will set your teen on a one-way road to academic failure. And you might be right. Or your teenager does need some help, but not nearly as much as you're used to providing.

Either way, the stage is set for a battle of wills that could end with no victor if your teen's academic performance becomes a casualty. Where can you turn to ensure a better outcome? Not always the teen's teachers, interestingly enough. Some teachers will suggest that the teen needs to manage her own academic requirements, that it is time for her to accept responsibility for her behavior, and that if she doesn't, she'll experience and learn from the negative consequences. Unfortunately, for students with executive skills deficits who may have a history of school performance problems, the negative consequences of school failure rarely teach a lesson or help the student succeed. You already know why if you've read much of this book: (1) the behavior management trick of using unpleasant consequences to discourage undesirable behavior won't work when it's not that the teen *won't* do what's required but that he *can't* because he doesn't have the necessary executive skills; and (2) executive skills deficits often come with an inability to recognize the relationship between a current behavior (for example, spending time on Facebook when there is a biology test tomorrow) and the consequences of that behavior (a poor grade on the test) or the longer-term consequences (poor grades interfering with college admission). So, left in a sink-or-swim dilemma, your teen may just sink.

This risk probably reinforces your belief that you need to continue to function as your teen's frontal lobes where schoolwork is concerned. But if your teen considers your involvement intrusive and agrees with any teachers who may think it's time for her to handle this responsibility on her own, she's not likely to be overly forthcoming with accurate and timely information, leaving you with nothing concrete to monitor. Who among us with teenage children having trouble in school hasn't had a conversation like this?

PARENT: I looked at PowerSchool online, and it looks like you have a biology assignment due. Where are you at with it?

STUDENT: The teacher gave us time to finish it in class.

> *or*

> I did it during my study period.

> *or*

> We didn't get through everything today, so she's going to give us an extra day.

> *or*

> I'm going over to Kendra's house to work on it.

You undoubtedly know from experience that any one of these statements may not be entirely accurate. So now you have to decide whether to take your inquiry to the next level and ask to see the assignment. If you do, you can expect resistance, possibly attacks on your lack of trust in your teen. And even if your teen does produce something, will you be confident that you know exactly what you are looking at?

The point is this: unless you are willing to expend considerable and sustained effort to monitor your teen's performance and you are able to tolerate

the likely pushback from your child, this is a difficult undertaking for a parent, particularly over the long term.

Fortunately, there is a potentially powerful alternative: coaching for the student with executive skills problems. What is a coach? Traditionally, a coach is a person who works with an athlete to help the athlete develop a set of skills and then apply those skills in a particular task or situation to achieve a positive outcome. Along the way, the coach monitors the athlete's skill acquisition, provides corrective feedback when needed, and offers encouragement. In our recent book for educators called *Coaching Students with Executive Skills Deficits*, we presented a model in which the person being coached is a student like your teen and the task or gain is academic performance. Essentially this approach is designed to help students learn executive skills and to establish a link between their hopes and dreams—their long-term goals—and what they will need to do on a daily basis to accomplish those long-term goals.

In the years since we first developed our coaching model, we have seen teenagers use the process to accomplish small, time-limited goals such as improving math homework completion and accuracy rates all the way to making the honor roll for the first time in high school as a stepping-stone to getting into a competitive college. Some of these results were achieved by us in the work we've done with students, but there have also been dissertations and published studies on the effective employment of our coaching model.

To test our model early on, we conducted a pilot study in a high school in New Hampshire. In this study, coaches worked with five students who through coaching were able to improve their grades significantly. For example, in the year before they worked with a coach, about 60% of the grades they were earning were C's. During the two marking periods in which they worked with a coach, over 60% of the grades they earned were B or better.

We see the coaching process as a bridge to help students like your teen strengthen the skills they will need when they may be stuck due to the realities of adolescence. If your teen has a history of not living up to his potential in school as a result of executive skills problems, his self-confidence is likely to have suffered some erosion. He may be understandably wary of investing a lot of himself in an enterprise that can produce another disappointment right at a time when academic demands are increasing. Simultaneously, pride may become an obstacle to accepting help from Mom or Dad. Together, these factors can lead to a continual downhill slide in academic performance.

Enter the coach: A good coach can help boost your teen's skills *and* confidence, in great part because this individual has just enough distance from your teen to avoid threatening the teen's pride or making the teen feel babied as she might when a parent tries to play this role during adolescence. Coaching is an ideal intervention for students who are underachievers due to weak executive skills but don't necessarily have a diagnosed disability, because a coach can pinpoint the one or two executive skills weaknesses that typically are standing between the student and academic achievement. Then the coach can help the teen find ways to strengthen those weaknesses or use her strengths to compensate for her shortcomings. The outcome: more consistent achievement of the high quality of work the teen is capable of. The bonus: renewed confidence and willingness to invest in academic effort.

In terms of the approaches to managing executive skills weaknesses outlined earlier in this book, the coach functions as both an environmental modification and a teacher of the skill. In those roles, the coach performs three critical functions:

1. Directly addresses a school achievement problem of concern to the student, parents, and teachers

2. Creates a buffer between parent and teen over an issue that typically leads to conflict

3. Plays the role of surrogate frontal lobe, whose influence is gradually reduced over time as the student becomes more proficient and practiced in using his or her executive skills

Sounds great, but how do you know whether coaching is the right way to go for your teen? In the rest of this chapter we'll answer the following questions, which should help you make an informed decision:

• What are the objectives of the coaching process?

• Who is and is not a candidate for coaching?

• How can you "sell" coaching to your teenager?

• How do you approach the school?

• Who will initiate the process?

• What characteristics should you look for in a coach, and how do you find one?

• How exactly does the coaching process work?

Objectives of the Coaching Process

We see coaching as having three major objectives. The first involves the coach and the student working together to establish long-term academic goals. This is an essential first step in helping to shift the student's focus away from the immediate satisfaction of day-to-day activities and toward some future hope or desire. The second objective is to help the student continuously understand the connection between day-to-day or even hour-to-hour tasks and behaviors and the student's longer-term goal. When students establish a long-term goal and appreciate how their day-to-day behavior and performance can impact that goal, they get one step closer to freeing themselves from the immediate temptations of the situation. The third objective of coaching is to have the student practice, on a day-to-day basis, the executive skills necessary to accomplish the short-term tasks that lead to achievement of the long-term goal. By building in a daily check-in procedure with the coach, the student begins to learn his pattern of strengths and weaknesses—which skills he can rely on to help and which weaknesses are an impediment to task completion.

Is Your Teen a Candidate for Coaching?

The teenagers we've worked with who respond best to coaching are those who believe they could be doing better in school than they are now, who recognize they have some shortcomings that are standing in the way of their doing better, and who are willing to work with someone to find ways to get around those shortcomings. It helps if they have some goal in mind that they want to work toward, even if it's just bringing up a grade or two on their report card or trying to be more consistent with homework completion. We've had some high school students find the idea of coaching attractive because it's a way to get their parents "off their backs," while others find it helpful to know that someone's going to be checking in with them to make sure they're following through on plans and goals.

Coaching is a collaborative process. The coach does not lay down the law and expect obedience from the student. The student participates in goal setting and in devising ways to reach the goals. Therefore motivation is critical, as is sufficient attentional capacity so that the student does not require recuing to task as often as every few minutes.

Although coaching, in our experience, is most effective with students of near average to average ability, this does not exclude students whose performance problems in school fall under different disability categories, as long as those disabilities are not extreme. For example, students with attention-deficit/hyperactivity disorder (ADHD) with mild to moderate attention problems whose impulsivity or distractibility is not extreme can benefit. Students with significant behavioral issues who have frequent discipline problems are not likely to be good candidates for coaching until these issues are resolved because they would have difficulty following through on the coaching procedures. On the other hand, students with Asperger syndrome have shown an ability to benefit from coaching, since they respond well to step-by-step procedures, are rule oriented, and are generally able to maintain good focus when they have a goal in mind. Finally, students with learning disabilities tend to respond well to coaching as long as the procedure is not seen as a substitute for more specifically addressing academic skill deficits.

Getting Your Teen to Buy In

To put it succinctly, coercion is not your best bet. Students need to agree voluntarily to participate in the coaching process if they're to get anything out of it, in the same way that athletes are coachable only when they want to play the sport. The coach is not responsible for chasing the student down, continuously confronting her, or imposing disciplinary consequences. If the coaching process is going to succeed, the relationship between coach and student must be one of collaboration and teamwork. If your teen's academic performance is poor but she is not committed to improving it, or if she insists she can handle the problem on her own, pressuring her into a coaching arrangement is likely to be futile.

This doesn't mean, however, that you shouldn't try to help your teen see the benefits he could gain. We always encourage parents and teachers to approach a reluctant student with specific information about what the process is, how it works, the choices the student has within the process, and the potential benefits to the student. At the end of this chapter you'll find a handout that you or your teen's teacher can give to your teen. The handout succinctly explains what the coaching process is about. We have seen reluctant students agree to participate in the long-term goal-setting process, since this involves no commitment other than to have a conversation with an adult and clearly focuses on eliciting information about what the student wants. Participating in this part of the coaching process may generate some interest in the student's moving further with it.

If, however, you and your teen are already embroiled in significant conflict over the teen's grades, you would be better off having the whole subject of coaching broached by a school staff member, such as a guidance counselor, who by definition is responsible for tracking student progress and interested in successful outcomes for the student.

If, in spite of these efforts, your teen is unwilling to try coaching, it's best not to push it. You or the guidance counselor can make it clear to the teen that the offer of coaching remains open should he change his mind in the future. Other options available to you are presented at the end of this chapter.

How to Approach the School

School counselors and school psychologists working in high schools are more informed about the impact of executive skills on school performance than they were in the past, and they need to be familiar with the concept of coaching. Some high schools and colleges already have coaching programs in place. But even if your teen's school does not, the counselors and psychologists are likely familiar enough with providing support systems to understand the rationale and what is required to implement coaching once they've read a description of the process.

We suggest you start by asking the high school guidance department if it provides a coaching service. If not, you may have to take the initiative, even to the point of providing resources to the school if the guidance counselors aren't familiar with the process.

In our experience, when students and parents initiate the process and the student is a willing participant, schools are quite willing to try to accommodate the student's needs. In fact, we've seen students who understood and were motivated to use the process approach a teacher or a high school staff person, describe the process, provide some resources to the teacher explaining how the procedure operates, and then begin the process with enthusiasm from the coach. Obviously, this demands a high level of initiative and motivation on the part of the student. For the student who has an initial conversation with the parent and agrees to consider coaching, another option is for the student alone or the student and parent together to approach the student's guidance counselor, describe the process, and solicit the counselor's help.

Selecting a Coach

Students who have had school performance problems as a result of executive skills weaknesses are likely to have heightened expectations of failure or underachievement, so it's important to find a coach your teen can trust and respect. The coaching process will require your teen to commit to a schedule of task completion that will be monitored on a frequent and regular basis, and because she won't always be successful, her coach needs to be someone she can tolerate being accountable to and being challenged by. Therefore, your teen should be active in the selection process and be able to identify the person she believes she can work with. In schools that have already established a formal coaching process, part of the procedure should involve matching so that the student and the coach feel comfortable with each other. In cases where the arrangement is more informal, we have found that students can identify high school staff they would be able to work with whom they respect and trust.

In a high school situation, any one of the following can fill the role:

- A favored teacher

- A paraprofessional

- A trained volunteer

- A staff intern

- A guidance counselor

- A special education teacher

- A school psychologist

- Another school employee (e.g., a secretary, assistant principal, nurse, etc.) that the student has established a connection with

It might even be another student, as long as there is an adult on staff who can supervise the coaching process.

Individuals who generally make good coaches have these characteristics:

- They are good listeners and empathic.

- They are reliable and have reasonably good planning skills.

- They like working with students and relate to them in a natural way.

- They teach through questions rather than lectures.

- They have had some training in coaching.

With regard to the last point, it has been our experience that high school staff who meet the other characteristics can obtain the training needed to coach by reading about the procedure in the resources provided at the end of the book, and, if possible, by checking in with another staff member who is familiar with the process during the first few sessions.

How the Coaching Process Works

There are basically two steps in the coaching process. In Step 1, the coach conducts a goal-setting session with the student. In Step 2, which is ongoing, the coach and the student meet for daily coaching sessions.

Step 1, the goal-setting session, involves three components:

1. The coach and the student set a goal. High school students are typically encouraged to set somewhat longer-term goals that may range from marking period grades to plans following high school completion.

2. With the coach's help, the student identifies potential obstacles that may stand in the way of achieving the goal as well as plans to overcome these obstacles.

3. The coach, based on the information provided by the student, writes out a plan for achieving the goal.

In Step 2, the daily coaching sessions, the purpose is to make a plan for the day. The objective of the coaching process is to help the student understand that the behaviors the student engages in on a daily basis impact the likelihood of her achieving the long-term goal. Daily coaching sessions can involve a number of questions:

1. Did the student complete the tasks that he said in yesterday's coaching session he would complete?

2. Was the student satisfied with the amount of effort and the product that resulted?

3. What work has been assigned today that needs to be completed for tomorrow?

4. When specifically will these tasks be completed, including the approximate amount of time needed?

5. Are there other activities that potentially interfere with work completion that need to be attended to?

6. Are there longer-term projects or tests that need to be planned for?

7. Is the student on target to meet her long-term goal?

When a student decides to participate in coaching, the extent to which parents participate in the process involves a negotiation among the student, the coach, and the parent. Since one of the reasons for (and a selling point of) coaching is to remove parents from a nagging role, it is important that parents respect the wishes of the student. At the same time, it is not likely that parents will or should abandon their interest or investment in their child's school performance; hence, we encourage parents to meet with the coach and the student at the beginning of the process to work out the details about how communication will take place, on what schedule, and what type of information will be communicated. Parents will continue to get detailed report information, and we recommend that a mechanism be built in so that a parent is contacted by the coach if the student is not participating in the process.

If Not Coaching, Then What?

In spite of your best efforts, your teen may not be interested in having a coach. When that's the case, you will need to play a more active role. Giving your teen the option of solving a problem first is generally the best approach, but the longer academic problems persist, and the more significant the decline in performance, the more likely it is that the teen will feel overwhelmed and unable to dig out from the problem. To prevent this, we recommend that you take the following steps:

• If the teen indicates that she will handle the problem herself, establish some short-term benchmarks as evidence that the problem is being addressed. "Short-term" depends partly on the type and significance of the problem. If it involves late or missing assignments, then we recommend weekly or biweekly feedback. If assignments and quizzes are being managed but test grades are weak, the feedback will be determined by the frequency with which tests are given.

• Establish a system for getting independent verification of progress. As a general rule, it should be at intervals shorter than report cards or progress reports. While teens may balk at this, relying on their assurance that the problem is being addressed, without feedback from teachers, is a risky proposition. If this is the first time that school performance problems have arisen, and you want to give your teen the benefit of the doubt, decide with the teen what the benchmark will be and when, other than at the time of the teen's reassurance, you will have information. This is most likely to be at the time of progress reports or report cards. Also agree on what the degree of improvement will be. For example, while going from a nearly failing grade to a barely passing grade is improvement, it may not be what you had in mind.

• If your teen can't deliver on his assurance, that at the very least, the next step in the process is short-term performance feedback provided by teachers. Many schools are now equipped with parent portals where student progress can be viewed almost in real time as long as teachers are up to date in their posting. If not, then we would recommend at least weekly e-mail contact with the teacher regarding specific performance.

• If the teen's good intentions plus frequent teacher feedback are not enough to resolve the problem, you will need to take a more active role. This means that you and your teen meet together with the teacher to hear the teacher's take on the problem, the teacher's suggestions for a solution, and the teen's reaction to this. The outcome of this meeting should be a plan of action with fairly quick feedback from the teacher about the success of the plan. If, from your perspective, a reasonable plan has been proposed and the teen balks, then it is time to consider the types of incentives and motivators presented in Chapter 5.

• If the process reaches this point, there is an increased likelihood of conflict between you and your teen. Considering the significant future consequences for a teen who is underperforming or failing in school, it is important to remain persistent and supportive in your efforts to help your teen resolve the problem.

Following is a brief description of the coaching process that you can photocopy and use to introduce the idea to your teen or to school staff members who are not already familiar with coaching.

An Overview of the Coaching Process

The coaching model has been designed to help teenagers be more success-ful in school and reach the career goals they set for themselves. The model has two phases: In Phase 1, the coach works with the student to develop a specific and realistic set of long-range goals and a plan for meeting those goals. In Phase 2, the coach works with the student on a regular basis to help the student plan his or her time, organize assignments, break down tasks, develop effective study skills, and, above all, to act as a supporter and advocate. A brief description of this process follows.

PHASE 1: LONG-TERM GOAL SETTING

Long-term goal setting with secondary-level students includes setting goals with respect to both high school graduation and post-high-school plans. If these plans include college, the coach works with the student to iden-tify what kind of college the student hopes to attend (for example, 2-year, 4-year, state university, liberal arts college). If the student wants to attend a particular college, this is included as part of the goal. The steps in Phase 1 are as follows:

- *Step 1:* The coach asks the student to describe his or her long-term goals and, if needed, helps the student refine them by asking clarifying questions: Do you plan to graduate from high school? Are you taking college, general, or vocational track classes? What do you hope to do after you finish high school—for example, continue with further school-ing or job training or get a job, and if so, what type of job would you hope to get?

- *Step 2:* Working with one goal at a time, the coach and the student determine what steps the student needs to take to achieve that goal. This may be as simple as getting passing grades in all classes, or it may be more complicated. It the student is applying to a competitive col-lege, for instance, goals may include making the honor roll, enrolling in honors-level or AP classes, participating in extracurricular activities, and the coach may need to discuss with the student the need to sign up for the kinds of classes required by the college that he or she is interested in.

- *Step 3:* The coach and the student discuss what obstacles will need to be overcome to achieve a particular goal. Many of these obstacles may involve specific behaviors such as choosing to do more interesting things

(cont.)

than homework, leaving assignments to the last minute with a resulting loss of quality, skipping classes, or forgetting to hand in homework.

- *Step 4:* The coach and the student discuss how the student can work
to overcome the obstacles that he or she has identified. For instance,
if leaving things until the last minute is an obstacle, the student might
decide that making and following a timeline for a long-term project
could help. If forgetting homework is a problem, developing a cuing
system to help remember homework might address this obstacle. The
coach and the student work together to identify one or two strategies
to address each obstacle.

- *Step 5:* At this point, the coach and the student work together to help
the student identify what environmental supports or modifications
need to be put in place to enhance the likelihood of success. This might
include test-taking modifications, such as extended time limits or taking
tests in a quiet room, access to tutorial services for weak subject areas,
a daily or weekly homework monitoring system to help the student stay
current with assignments, assistance with time management or organizational skills, or a homework incentive system.

- *Step 6:* The last step in the session is for the coach to check with the
student one last time to ensure that the plan being developed is realistic and within the capabilities of the student to achieve. Although plans
can be revised as necessary as coaching continues, every effort should
be made to develop a plan at the outset that has a reasonable chance
of success.

PHASE 2: DAILY COACHING SESSIONS

The purpose of the daily coaching session is primarily for the coach to help
the student plan what tasks he or she has to accomplish before the next
coaching session and to identify when the task will be completed. With the
exception of the very first daily session, each session follows the same format by using the acronym REAP (Review, Evaluate, Anticipate, Plan).

In the first session the coach and student *Review* the results of the long-
range goal-setting session. The coach may begin with a question such as
"What was it we talked about when we met before?" or "Tell me what you
remember about the goals you set at our last meeting." Although notes from
the long-range goal-setting session can be referred to, the student begins
by answering this question based on his or her recollection of that meeting. The session then moves toward a discussion of immediate tasks and

(*cont.*)

responsibilities, beginning with an overview of whatever longer-term obligations the student might have, including schoolwork as well as extracurricular responsibilities (sports activities, jobs, clubs, etc.).

The coach then asks the student to identify what the student hopes to accomplish before the next coaching session. This is written down (by the coach) and includes all academic tasks, both homework due the next day and long-term projects that need to be started or upcoming tests and quizzes that need to be studied for. Here the coach and the student may work together on developing timelines and setting reasonable study goals for tests. The student may also want to work on behavioral goals (for example, "answer more questions in Spanish class" or "stay after school for extra help in biology"). Once specific tasks are identified, the coach has the student say when he or she plans to do each task. The coach gets the student to be as specific as possible about when the task will be accomplished (for example, "during eighth-period study hall" or "between 7:00 and 8:00 P.M. this evening"). The meeting concludes with a brief assessment of how the session went. Both the coach and the student have a copy of the written plan to take away from the session.

All subsequent sessions begin with a review of the tasks identified at the previous coaching session to determine whether the plans were carried out as intended. Referring to the plan completed at the previous session, the coach reads each item on the list and asks if the student did the task. The student is then asked to rate *(Evaluate)* how well he or she accomplished the task, perhaps using a rating scale. This is followed by a brief discussion between the coach and the student about the goals set and the student's performance.

The next step is to have the student *Anticipate* work that he or she has to do in the near future. Now a new plan is developed. This may mean transferring relevant information from the previous plan and adding in the new assignments, tests, or responsibilities that may have come up since the previous session. The final step, as in the first session, is for the coach and student to work together to *Plan* what will be done before the next coaching session.

Particularly in the early stages of the coaching process, the emphasis by the coach is on support. If the coach notes that the student frequently fails to follow through on the plans he or she has devised, they work together to evaluate where the plans are breaking down, but the coach also may want to help the student revise the plan or long-term goal to make it more realistic and achievable. As time goes on and the student and coach become more comfortable working with each other, the coach may be more direct in challenging the student to accomplish daily tasks.

21

....

Transitions

If you look back on your teen's elementary and middle school years, you'll be reminded of what a huge transition high school has represented for your son or daughter. Adolescents are exposed to new peer groups, different teachers, the opportunity to earn their own money, and driving. They have a variety of choices for extracurricular activities and growing opportunities to move more freely about their environment. They also understand that independence in the form of legal decision making is within sight, and every aspect of their culture encourages them to establish an identity for themselves. They are well on the road to a transition that will largely remove them from the personal and institutional supports that they have had since birth, namely transition to college or to a job and independent living.

As a parent, this period in your teen's life gives you a clear view of the possibilities and the pitfalls and the realization that you have a limited amount of time to help your teen prepare for these next major transitions. Throughout this book, we have tried to provide you with the means to understand the strengths and weaknesses of your teen's executive skills and strategies for how best to prepare the teen for the next phases in life. At the same time, you have probably come to realize that teens with significant executive skills weaknesses represent a work in progress for parents. Thus transitions toward adulthood do not signal the end of that work. In fact, while some aspects of parental support will end, if only because of the lack of proximity of parent to child, others will need to continue. These include emotional and financial support and continued advice and guidance. The same is true for educational supports. The type of support and the way in which it is provided will be dictated in part by the nature of the executive skills weakness and how it manifests itself in day-to-day living, as well as by the type of support that the teen is willing to accept.

To make this discussion more concrete, let's consider transitions that both teens and parents have a significant investment in—going on to college after high school, or to a job and independent living. Our focus here is on the teen whose executive skill weaknesses represent the most significant risk for failure. We have referred elsewhere in this book to "context-dependent" teens. These are the teens whose behavior is more likely to be influenced by an immediate or near-term payoff than by a long-term goal. These teens may in fact have a long-term goal—in this case, college or a job—and be sincere in their desire and intent to achieve this goal. However, they lose sight at times of the path that connects their current behavior to the long-term goal and may struggle to get to it. Behaviorally, with context-dependent teens, parents see the following characteristics:

- Instead of working on a project, they are likely to go on Facebook or surf the Internet.

- They are susceptible to peer influences to the extent that they could get or perhaps have already gotten into trouble.

- You are reluctant to leave them unsupervised at home on weekend nights.

- They routinely underestimate the amount of time that school tasks or chores will take, and as a result have late or missing assignments or fail to complete chores on a regular basis.

- They know when job or college applications are due but still need to be prodded constantly by you to get them in on time.

From an assessment perspective, teens with context-dependent behavior tend to show weaknesses in the following executive skills areas: time management, task initiation, sustained attention, and goal-directed persistence. When they are in high school, teens with this constellation of weaknesses may, as a result of concerted efforts by parents and teachers, perform well enough to accomplish their goal. They are the teens who parents and teachers feel might have done significantly better (for example, obtained scholarships, been accepted at more challenging colleges, gotten better jobs) if they had made more "effort" or been "more focused."

Off to College

Let's start with transitions to college. For students with this constellation of executive skills weaknesses, while getting into college is a laudable accomplishment, it may signal the beginning rather than the end of a problem. That's because in making this transition the teen is moving from an environment where there was a significant level of support to a new environment where there are few if any such supports. While it may not seem so to you, teens who are living at home with curfews, school attendance and grade expectations, and behavior monitoring actually have a fairly supportive environment. Contrast this with college, when your teen moves away. Moment-to-moment supervision ranges from minimal to nonexistent. No one will provide cues regarding curfews, wake-up times, and so forth. There will be no immediate repercussions if your teen does not attend class or complete assignments. And, college and community rules notwithstanding, mood- and behavior-altering substances are readily available. In this type of situation, the context-dependent teen is the proverbial kid in a candy store. When the various supports that were part of the naturally occurring environment are not available, there is a reasonably good chance that the immediate context and the availability of more immediate gratification will have a significant impact on behavior. All students who transition from high school to college are subject to these influences, and changes in behavior are likely even for the most focused of students. However, the majority of teens who make this transition do so successfully, based on their continuing to have a long-term goal and an appreciation that getting to class and completing assignments on a regular basis is the path to accomplishing that goal. Parents contribute to this goal-directed persistence while monitoring performance from a distance, and their children know they can only continue to enjoy the freedom afforded by college if their performance is acceptable.

Is your teen likely to struggle in the transition to college? We have developed a set of questions that you can ask yourself by the end of the second or third marking term of senior year:

1. Can your teen wake up on his own and get to school on time at least 90% of the time?

2. Can your teen keep track of homework assignments without a lot of monitoring from you?

3. Does your teen recognize that she has some executive skills weaknesses that may interfere with school performance, and has she put systems in place to address these—for example, reminders for due dates, ways of using friends as cuing mechanisms or study buddies, organizational systems for keeping track of materials?

4. Can your teen manage competing distractions so they don't significantly interfere with school or other obligations? In other words, can he set aside preferred activities to complete nonpreferred activities with some degree of responsibility (this does not mean the student is gunning to be an A student, but is he realistic about how much work it takes to earn grades that are acceptable to both him and his parents?).

5. If the student doesn't quite pull off any of the above to your satisfaction, are there any other signs that the student is willing to work hard to achieve personal goals, such as following a rigorous sports schedule, holding down a job that includes some responsibilities, or pursuing other hobbies or interests to produce a product or achieve a desired tangible result?

6. Can your teen make responsible choices when temptation presents itself? Can your teen stand up to peers when they suggest doing something risky or illegal?

7. Does the student really, really, really want to go to college, or is she going through the motions to please you?

If, based on your experience with your teen in high school, you have reason to be concerned about his ability for self-regulation of behavior and goal-directed persistence in a new environment, you have a number of options to help ensure that your teen stays on track. These include:

• Monitor course requirements, completion of assignments, and grades if possible. Many college professors post the course syllabus, due dates, and grades during the semester, and you can access this information with your child's permission by logging on to the website. If in advance of the time your child leaves for college you have discussed expectations for performance or even specific grades, monitoring and periodic conversations about performance may be sufficient to help the teen stay on track. If you used a system like this in high school and your child benefited from it, you can continue to use it. These systems require a fair amount of work and a fair amount of tolerance from your child.

• Set some expectations about grades and tie this to continuing tuition support. Be sure, however, to take into account the fact that your teen is making a significant transition to a new environment and needs a period of adjustment. These also may need to be adjusted during the term, since performance will vary with course difficulty. On the other hand, you are likely to have sufficient information about your child's ability level and performance capabilities to establish a reasonable set of expectations. Studies looking at the amount of time that college students, on average, study suggest that few of them are in danger of stress-related illnesses as a result of weekly study schedules.

• If your teen's performance in the past suggests that she requires ongoing monitoring, consider getting a coach at school. The functions of coaching described in Chapter 20 for high school should be similar at the college level. Most colleges offer tutorial support as part of their student services, and increasing numbers of colleges are familiar with the notion of coaching to provide help with organization, time management, and task initiation through regular check-ins.

• Enlist aid from the student support services at school. It is in the best interest of colleges to retain their students, and virtually all of them offer a range of services to assist students negotiating college. An increasing number of schools are routinely offering, or in some cases requiring, freshmen to avail themselves of courses as a kind of extended orientation to college. (This is Dick talking:) At my daughter's school, the freshman course was University 101 and included information on study skills, time management, and academic support as well as how to manage the distractions of college life.

• If you have concerns about your teen's commitment to college, have him contribute to his tuition. Since most teens enter college with few resources of their own, this will probably have to be through loans. You can create an incentive for improved performance by agreeing to pay off part of the loan contingent on his achieving a particular grade point average. Simply having "skin in the game" adds an incentive to performance.

• If you are concerned about your student's ability to handle the demands of college work, have her enroll in a college course during the summer of her junior or senior year. Many universities now offer this option to high school students, and it is an effective way for parents and teens to understand the demands and expectations of college courses.

• Have your student take a reduced course load. At most universities, 12 credits are still considered to be full-time. If reduced course loads are taken on an ongoing basis, a 4-year education becomes a 5-year education with potentially significant increases in cost. However, if the objective is to do this for one or two semesters as a way for the student to acclimate to college, it can be an effective temporary solution.

• Have the student live at home. We have worked with families for whom this has been an effective college introduction for the student. It is, in effect, a postgraduate year with some of the same supports in place but at a higher level of demand. In difficult economic times, it can be an attractive option and an effective way to assess a student's readiness for college.

• Have the student take a year (or more) off. Let's remember that we are talking about maturation of the frontal lobes and corresponding development of executive skills. Giving students the opportunity to take some time off and earn some money can change their perspective about school and have a positive impact on their work ethic when they do enroll.

• Remember that college is not the only option. We have, unfortunately, been indoctrinated into the notion that a college education is the minimum requirement for success in our society. In fact, companies and employers are interested in individuals who have skills that fit with that company's needs. College is not the only way to obtain these skills, and in some cases they are better obtained through vocational technical schools, apprenticeships, and on-the-job training programs.

Independent Living

That point brings us to the second possible transition—a job and independent living. Let's start with the independent living piece. In this culture at this time in history, given this economy, there's a pretty good chance that your teen won't move out after high school. (In fact, most college grads are now moving back home.) If that's the case, you and your teen need to settle a number of issues, including but not limited to the following:

• Assuming he gets a job, should he pay room and board, or should he be asked to set aside money in a savings account to help him prepare for the day when he will move out?

• Do you expect him to tell you where he is at night and when he will be coming home?

- Can he have his girlfriend spend the night in his bedroom?

- Can he sleep until noon every day?

- Can he drive your car and not fill it up with gas on his dime?

- Can he spend all hours of the day and night playing video games? Or practicing with his band in your garage?

You get the point. If your child is living at home and out of school, issues need to be discussed, negotiated, and resolved at the beginning of the arrangement and not when you begin to get on each other's nerves.

Jobs

Next comes the job issue and the questions that must be settled, some of which are intertwined with the living issue:

- Is it reasonable to expect that your child will get a job if he's not going to college? (This is not as self-evident to teens as you might think.)

- If she can't find a job, what is it reasonable for you to expect her to be doing (for example, some combination of job-seeking activities and participating in household maintenance by doing chores)?

- If you expect him to help out at home, do you pay him?

- If she gets a job in a distant city but it's not enough to pay the rent, should you be willing to help out?

- How much should you help out? For how long?

- What if it's an unpaid internship or apprenticeship?

- What if your teen's friend gets a job and wants to share an apartment with him even though he doesn't have a job? Should you support that?

Our intent here is not to present a comprehensive list of all the questions that may arise but rather to give you a flavor of what potential areas of concern are.

As with all of the other issues we have discussed, the key point here is to have an open discussion with your adolescent about your concerns, what the costs are, what you can provide, and what your child thinks of certain scenarios that may take shape. We believe it is critical to have this discussion well before a student leaves if she is going to college. If she is not, then you and your child will still save yourselves a great deal of aggravation by resolving as many of the questions above as possible. In either case, it is important to specifically discuss different possibilities so that you and your teen anticipate what may happen and know how the issue will be managed.

Fast-Forward

Looking down the road at some of the stories from earlier chapters:

Remember Stephanie and Nick? Nick had a working memory deficit that caused him to miss a dentist appointment, leading his organized and distraught mother to the breaking point. They solved the problem by getting Nick a smartphone. Three years later Nick (now a freshman in college) and Stephanie agree that he has made improvements. It took time and patience, but Nick adheres to his phone's calendar and has trained himself to automatically enter new appointments at the exact time that he makes them. Stephanie still sees room for improvement, though. Nick has gotten markedly better at reminding himself of events, but paper deadlines and commitments made offhandedly are still frequently overlooked. Stephanie is concerned that this will become a serious roadblock when it comes to meeting due dates for his work in college, especially when he gets into his major. Nick needs to apply for either an internship or a summer job, and he has trouble adhering to his own deadlines unless they are tied to a specific outside authority. His mother wishes Nick could develop a system of more general reminders, like "on or before this date, I need to have recommendation letters from the following professors." Stephanie hopes that Nick will learn to take his own to-do lists as seriously as his commitments to other people.

Or what about Brian and Bella, two of our cases that involved driving? Brian got into a minor car accident due to being distracted, and Bella was an impulsive speeder who was pulled over by the police. Well, 2 years later, both are back behind the wheel. Brian took his insurance deductible out of his work check, and Bella worked off her speeding ticket by digging and planting some new garden beds under the close supervision of her mom. Now Brian uses a cell phone application that hides all incoming texts and calls while he's driving. This solution involves a level of trust between him and his parents, but thus far his driving has been incident free. He has his own car, but since they still cover his insurance, his parents' concern is that when he moves out of the house and doesn't have them around as a constant reminder, he will lapse into his old habits.

Bella was allowed back on the road but was relegated to use of only her father's station wagon, and to this day the coupe is off limits. Now Bella wants to buy her own car, and while she has a job, it's clear that she'll need financial assistance from her parents. They have agreed to help her, on one condition involving a recent innovation from the car insurance companies. Bella will have to install a device in her car that constantly monitors her driving habits. If she adheres to the rules of the road, it will record this. Over time, Bella could actually see reductions in her insurance payments from consistently responsible road behavior. Since her parents have agreed to contribute a flat amount to her insurance payments, good driving doesn't just please her parents; it's also lucrative for Bella to be safe when behind the wheel.

Finally, what about Brad, whose mom, Kathy, was having daily shouting matches with him and felt like her home had become a war zone because of Brad's hostile attitude? While things have since improved on the home front, Kathy and Mark (Brad's father) are very concerned about how Brad will behave now that he's in a college setting, specifically with roommates who won't be so tolerant or understanding when Brad's temper flares. They have discussed the issue with Brad, and he has come up with a few ideas. During orientation, they heard about the dispute mediation program run by the university housing office, and Brad says he is willing to use this if the need arises. He plans to familiarize himself with the common areas in the dorm and make friends besides his roommates. He sees this as a way to provide himself with physical separation from his roommates if necessary and to avoid feeling as though he is trapped in his room during a conflict. Mark and Kathy know that only time will tell, but for now they are incredibly proud of the thoughtfulness and initiative of their son. There are bound to be fights down the road; some just cannot be avoided. But they are confident that their son is conscious of his weakness, and his coming up with a plan himself reassures them that he is prepared to solve the problems that any college student encounters.

We offer these examples as a reminder that kids with executive skills weaknesses are a work in progress. Reaching "legal age" and heading off to college or to a job do not guarantee that they are past the need for your support or help. Nonetheless, if you've gotten to this point and have successfully navigated most of the adolescent storms, you have a good idea of your teen's strengths and weaknesses and the strategies that have been most effective. This experience sets the tone for your role in the next phase of your teen's life. You'll be less involved on a day-to-day basis, and when it comes to help and support, you'll follow the teen's lead. This does not mean that you accommodate every request, but as much as possible you honor those that point to self-sufficiency. Ultimately, your success is defined by the extent to which you've worked yourself out of your job as a parent.

Resources

Books

Barkley, R. A. (1997). *ADHD and the Nature of Self-Control.* New York: Guilford Press.—This book is fairly technical, but it provides a good description of executive skills within a developmental framework and argues that executive skills are at the core of ADHD. Russell Barkley has written a number of other books that parents may find helpful, especially parents of defiant children or those with ADHD. These include:

- *Taking Charge of ADHD: The Complete, Authoritative Guide for Parents.*
- *Your Defiant Teen: 10 Steps to Resolve Conflict and Rebuild Your Relationship* (coauthored by Arthur Robin).

In addition, Barkley's *Taking Charge of Adult ADHD* (Guilford, 2010) is filled with practical suggestions that many teens will be able to use for managing all areas of life, from school and work to money, driving, health, and more.

Bradley, M. J. (2002). *Yes, Your Teen is Crazy!: Loving Your Kid without Losing Your Mind.* Gig Harbor, WA.: Harbor Press.—In this humorous, blunt book Bradley puts adolescent behaviors that seem "nuts" in the context of brain development and reassures parents that they still have an important and influential role in their teens' lives and that they have important responsibilities and need to set expectations for teen behavior.

Dawson, P., & Guare, R. (2009). *Smart but Scattered: The Revolutionary "Executive Skills" Approach to Helping Kids Reach Their Potential.* New York: Guilford Press.— This book is written primarily for parents of children from ages 4 to 14 and professionals who work with them. The book describes how executive skills develop, how to evaluate strengths and weaknesses, and how parents can help their children develop these skills.

Dawson, P., & Guare, R. (2010). *Executive Skills in Children and Adolescents: A Practical*

275

Guide to Assessment and Intervention (2nd ed.). New York: Guilford Press.—This book, written primarily for educators and school psychologists, describes how executive skills are assessed but also provides descriptions of school-based interventions for executive skills weaknesses following the same framework that the authors describe in the current volume.

Dawson, P., & Guare, R. (2012). *Coaching Students with Executive Skills Deficits*. New York: Guilford Press.—This manual presents an evidence-based coaching model for helping students whose academic performance or behavior is suffering due to weaknesses in executive skills.

Faber, A., & Mazlish, E. (2006). *How to Talk So Teens Will Listen and Listen So Teens Will Talk*. New York: William Morrow.—This book reassures you that the experiences you're going through with your teen are shared by most parents of teens. A willingness to communicate and share openly combined with high expectations and predictable structure will serve both you and your teen well.

Feinstein, S. (2009). *Inside the Teenage Brain: Parenting a Work in Progress* (2nd ed). Lanham, MD: R & L Education.—Feinstein's book focuses on the relationship between adolescent brain development and the unique behaviors of teens. She also distinguishes between parenting styles that work (trust, support, balanced communication) and those that don't (arguing, lecturing, and nagging).

Goldberg, E. (2001). *The Executive Brain: Frontal Lobes and the Civilized Mind*. New York: Oxford University Press.—A somewhat technical but very readable description of how the frontal lobes of the brain control judgment and decision making. For people who want a more thorough description of research delineating executive skills, this is an excellent resource.

Greene, R. (2010). *The Explosive Child: A New Approach for Understanding and Parenting Easily Frustrated, Chronically Inflexible Children* (rev. ed.). This very readable book is a source of comfort to parents of inflexible children, as it describes the causes of inflexibility as well as ways to treat the problem in clear, straightforward language.

Harvey, V. S., & Chickie-Wolfe, L. A. (2007). *Fostering Independent Learning: Practical Strategies to Promote Student Success*. New York: Guilford Press.—This book, written primarily for educators and school psychologists, describes strategies to help students become independent learners. There is considerable overlap with the concepts described in our book, and parents may be able to use some of the strategies described by Harvey and Chickie-Wolfe.

Kastner, L. S., & Wyatt, J. (2009). *Getting to Calm: Cool-Headed Strategies for Parenting Tweens and Teens*. Seattle, WA: Parent Map.—With new brain research in adolescents as a path to connecting with teens, the authors lead parents through strategies to work through issues from rude comments to lying and substance abuse. They offer clear suggestions for communication to maintain loving relationships while at the same time setting limits.

Levine, M. (2002). *A Mind at a Time*. New York: Simon & Schuster.—Mel Levine has written many books parents may find helpful. We like this one the best. Here, he describes eight different brain "systems," the roles they play in learning, and how parents and teachers can take advantage of learning strengths and bypass weaknesses to help children be successful students. A PBS documentary describes Dr. Levine's work (available at *www.pbs.org/wgbh/misunderstoodminds*).

Maitland, T. E., & Quinn, P. O. (2010). *Ready for Take-Off: Preparing Your Teen with ADHD or LD for College.* Washington, DC: Magination.—Maitland and Quinn address a critical issue in this book that directly applies to students with executive skills deficits: successfully making the transition to a college environment where fewer supports will be available. Parents can increase the likelihood of success by using a "coaching-style" approach to enhance their teen's self-management skills.

Martin, C., Dawson, P., & Guare, R. (2007). *Smarts: Are We Hardwired for Success?* New York: AMACOM.—This book applies our executive skills construct to an adult population, particularly focusing on workplace issues and how people can take advantage of their executive skills strengths and work around their weaknesses to function more effectively on the job.

Phelan, T. J. (2012). *Surviving Your Adolescents: How to Manage—and Let Go of—Your 13–18 Year Olds* (3rd ed.). Glen Ellyn, IL: ParentMagic.—The latest edition of Phelan's popular and encouraging book helps parents of teens learn to communicate and understand when and how to manage risks, when to let go, and when to seek professional help.

Quinn, P. O., & Maitland, T. E. (2011). *On Your Own: A College Readiness Guide for Teens with ADHD.* Washington, DC: Magination.—In this book, Quinn and Maitland provide specific information on the challenges that students face in the transition to college and more independent living, as well as concrete strategies for teens and their parents on how to prepare to these challenges. Much of the valuable information they present directly addresses how to improve executive skills.

Riera, M. (2003). *Staying Connected to Your Teenager: How to Keep Them Talking to You and How to Hear What They're Really Saying.* Cambridge, MA: Da Capo Press.—Riera looks at teens as having two very different personalities—one a regressed child and the other an emerging adult. He encourages parents to focus on the adult rather than the child and offers strategies to coax out the adult personality.

Schaefer, C. E., & DiGeronimo, T. F. (2000). *Ages & Stages: A Parent's Guide to Normal Childhood Development.* New York: Wiley.—This book provides an excellent parental guide to normal child development and includes, according to its authors, "tips and techniques for building your child's social, emotional, interpersonal, and cognitive skills."

Walsh, D. (2005). *WHY Do They Act That Way?: A Survival Guide to the Adolescent Brain for You and Your Teen.* New York: Free Press.—This book provides a detailed description of changes in the adolescent brain and how these changes help us understand teen behavior, as well as suggestions for parents on how to use this information to relate to their children.

Wolf, A. E. (2011). *I'd Listen to My Parents If They'd Just Shut Up: What to Say and Not Say When Parenting Teens.* New York: William Morrow.—Why is it that the simplest conversation with a teen can turn into a war of words? Wolf helps parents understand the sources of teens' "attitudes" and, more important, how to communicate to make parenting a teen a more enjoyable experience. Using specific scenarios, he identifies which communication strategies will work and which will fail.

Magazines

ADDitude is a magazine for families affected by ADHD. Every issue includes articles on a range of topics, many of which relate to executive skills, including product reviews, practical advice, and helpful suggestions for managing ADHD in both children and adults. They also offer a helpful website (*www.additudemag.com*).

ATTENTION! is the official publication of CHADD (Children and Adults with Attention Deficit/Hyperactivity Disorder). It serves the same audience served by *ADDitude* and contains similar practical articles. They, too, have a useful website (*www.chadd.org*).

Parents magazine offers general advice on child development and parenting issues. Their website is *www.parents.com*.

Organizations Offering Parenting Information and Support, Information on Adolescent Development, and Help for Disorders Associated with Executive Skills Deficits

About Kids Health (*www.aboutkidshealth.ca*), developed by the Hospital for Sick Children in Toronto, is a valuable source of information on topics involving child health, behavior, and development. The series on executive skills in children, including information on teens, is excellent.

American Academy of Pediatrics (*www.aap.org*) is the official website of the American Academy of Pediatrics. An excellent source of information about all aspects of children's and teenagers' health.

Autism Society Canada (*www.autismsocietycanada.ca*) is committed to advocacy, public education, information and referral, and provincial development support.

Autism Society of America (*www.autism-society.org*) is a national grassroots organization dedicated to promoting advocacy, education, support, services, and research for individuals on the autism spectrum including those with Asperger syndrome. Provides reliable, up-to-date information about autism spectrum disorders.

Autism Today (*www.canadianautism.com*) is a free membership organization that offers access to over 5,000 articles and other resources and a store for purchasing books and additional tools on autism spectrum disorders. The organization also plans workshops and conferences to disseminate information and practical advice about autism spectrum disorders.

Brain Connection (*www.brainconnection.com*) provides a variety of articles and resources for parents and professionals about brain development and new brain research, particularly as these relate to children's and teenagers' learning.

Canadian Paediatric Society (*www.cps.ca*) serves both CPS members and other health care professionals with information they need to make informed decisions about child and adolescent health care. Includes a page of resources on adolescent health under "children's health topics." Parents, journalists, and others involved in the care of children will also find the site useful.

CanChild Centre for Childhood Disability Research (*www.canchild.ca*) is a research and educational center. The majority of its research work is focused on issues that make a difference for children and teenagers with physical, developmental, and communication needs and their families.

Casey Life Skills (*www.caseylifeskills.org*) provides a detailed assessment for a broad range of adolescent life skills as well as resources for how parents and teens can acquire or strengthen these skills. It is the most comprehensive assessment we have seen of the skills that will be needed for independent adult living. It was designed for teens in foster care, but the skills are applicable to all teens. The assessment is free.

CHADD (*www.chadd.org*) is an organization dedicated to providing advocacy, education, and support for individuals with ADHD. The website is an excellent source of information for individuals, parents, and professionals about topics related to ADHD.

Children's Technology Review (*http://childrenstech.com*) provides professional reviews of interactive technology (software, video games) to help guide parents and professionals in monitoring and choosing products that children and teens are exposed to daily.

Council for Exceptional Children (*www.cec.sped.org*) is an international professional organization whose mission is to improve educational outcomes for students with disabilities and/or gifts and talents.

Family Education (*www.familyeducation.com*) is a website that's packed with information, parenting tips, and family games and activities aimed at parents of children from birth to age 18.

Gray Center for Social Learning and Understanding (*www.thegraycenter.org*) is devoted to promoting understanding between individuals on the autism spectrum and those who work alongside them. The site is an excellent source of information about the Social Stories approach, which parents and professionals can use as a teaching tool with all children.

Intervention Central (*www.interventioncentral.org*) offers a wide range of tools and resources that parents and school staffs can use to promote effective learning and positive classroom behavior for children.

Learning Disabilities Association of America (*www.ldanatl.org*) is an organization dedicated to promoting an understanding of learning disabilities, creating success for individuals affected by them, and reducing the incidence of these disabilities in the future. This is a comprehensive site for information about all aspects of learning disabilities.

Learning Disabilities Association of Canada (*www.ldac-acta.ca*) is a private nonprofit organization, composed mostly of parents but also professionals, whose mission is to serve as Canada's national voice for individuals with learning disabilities and those who support them. The association publishes books and other materials containing a broad range of helpful information and news in the field, and the site contains numerous links to other organizations in Canada and worldwide, as well as publications and legal assistance.

MyADHD (*www.myadhd.com*) is a subscription website that offers tools for assessment, treatment, and progress monitoring, as well as a library of articles, audio programs, and charts that parents can use to better understand and manage their teen's attention disorder.

National Autistic Society, United Kingdom (*www.nas.org.uk*) is a nonprofit parents' organization dedicated to providing a wide range of services and information for British families with children diagnosed with an autism spectrum disorder, from schools and outreach services to social and respite support, research data, diagnostic and treatment information, and parent courses and training. Based in London, the society has chapters throughout the United Kingdom and offers numerous resources for parents of adolescents.

National Center for Learning Disabilities (*www.ncld.org*) is a parent-led organization that promotes research and programs to facilitate effective learning, advocates for educational rights and opportunities, and provides information to parents, professionals, and individuals with learning disabilities.

National Institutes of Child Health and Human Development (NICHD) (*www.nichd.nih.gov*) supports and conducts research and clinical work on the neurobiological, developmental, and behavioral processes that affect children and families. Provides authoritative information about a broad range of child and adolescent health and behavioral issues.

PBS (*www.pbs.org*) has provided and continues to provide excellent, scientifically based programming on child health and development, including brain–behavior relationships.

PTA (*www.pta.org*) provides parents with extensive information and resources about topics such as student achievement, safety, media technology, nutrition, and health and wellness.

Psychiatric Times (*www.psychiatrictimes.com*) is an authoritative monthly online publication offering feature articles, clinical news, and reports on special topics across a broad range of psychiatric issues involving children and adults.

Raising Children Network (*http://raisingchildren.net.au*) is a comprehensive website for parents in Australia that includes resources, discussion forums, videos, and more, including information on teen development, learning difficulties, autism, and ADHD. Articles are keyed by age and therefore can be read by both parents and teens.

Specific Learning Disabilities Federation (SPELD) New Zealand (*www.speld.org.nz*) is a nonprofit advocacy organization dedicated to those with learning disabilities, including LDs associated with attention disorders and autism spectrum disorders, via chapters throughout New Zealand. The federation's main objectives are advocacy, assessment and tutoring, and family support. It offers courses and certification to train teachers and parents as learning disabilities tutors.

Thanet ADDers (*www.adders.org*) is a support resource based in Kent, England, and founded by a parent of an adult diagnosed with ADD who also has the disorder herself. The site offers support and information, links for buying books and other resources, and provides "as much free practical help" as possible to those dealing with ADD and ADHD.

Wrightslaw (*www.wrightslaw.com*) contains articles focusing on special education law and advocating for children with disabilities.

Websites Offering Additional Information on Specific Teen Issues Discussed in This Book

Driving

www.driveincontrol.com offers the nation's first state-certified crash prevention training to teens and drivers of other ages. The closed-course, hands-on education was adapted from existing law enforcement training in the United States as well as European instruction that led to a societal shift in attitudes toward driving in many countries.

www.skidschool.us offers training in reacting skillfully to unexpected driving conditions and emergencies at several training centers in New England.

www.driving-school.com/skid_training.php presents a specific skid-training course offered by Defensive Driving School, a driving school with a long history in the state of Washington.

www.safeteendrivingclub.org offers car data monitoring products as well as information on choosing a safe car for a teen and much more.

http://iihs.org, the website of the Insurance Institute for Highway Safety, can help you determine how safe your car or any other car your teen might end up driving is.

www.safercar.gov, the website of the National Highway Traffic Safety Administration (NHTSA), provides safety ratings (one to five stars) that you can use to evaluate your existing car or one you're considering buying for your teen to drive.

www.getizup.com offers a product that prevents cell phone usage while a car is in motion, discouraging distracted driving by teens.

Financial Management

www.cardratings.com is a site filled with information on the best credit cards and credit card terminology, credit card calculators, and the terms (in a database) of dozens of credit cards currently offered. Teens can learn how to use credit cards wisely by reading the articles on the site.

www.cajumpstart.org is the website of the California JumpStart Coalition, a non-profit organization dedicated to improving the personal financial education of the state's youth. Teens nationwide can access articles, surveys, studies, and more. Many resources are offered for teachers as well.

www.themint.org is a collaborative effort of the Northwestern Mutual Foundation, the charitable arm of Northwestern Mutual, and the National Council on Economic Education (NCEE) to help children and teens learn to manage money. There are tips and puzzles for children, teens, parents, and teachers that make money management engaging to learn.

Study and Homework Tips

www.childdevelopmentinfo.com, the website of the Child Development Institute, contains a wealth of resources for children with problems related to executive skills deficits. "Homework and study habits" in the dropdown list under "Learning" offers a lot of help for teens who need help with studying.

http://homeworktips.about.com offers links to numerous articles providing homework and book report tips, common test-taking errors, and using planners.

Index

About the Authors

Richard Guare, PhD, is Director of the Center for Learning and Attention Disorders in Portsmouth, New Hampshire, where **Peg Dawson, EdD,** works as a clinical school psychologist. With over 30 years of clinical experience, Drs. Dawson and Guare are coauthors of the best-selling *Smart but Scattered*, which focuses on younger children and preteens. **Colin Guare,** a 25-year-old freelance writer who grew up with an attention disorder, has contributed to *ADDitude* magazine and has worked with children with learning disorders.